Feeding Problems in Children

Edited by

Angela Southall
and
Anthony Schwartz

RADCLIFFE MEDICAL PRESS

Radcliffe Medical Press
18 Marcham Road, Abingdon, Oxon OX14 1AA

British Library Cataloguing in Publication Data

A catalogue record for this book is available from the British Library.

ISBN 1 85775 208 2

Typeset by Joshua Associates Ltd, Oxford
Printed and bound by TJ International Ltd, Padstow, Cornwall

Contents

Preface

Feeding is a fundamental process, essential to survival. The taking of food serves an important biological function, enabling the child to grow and develop both physically and psychologically. Feeding and eating have important psychosocial functions, too. From the onset, feeding experiences are central to the development of relationships with the primary care-givers, especially the mother. Later, eating forms an important and integral part of family and wider social interaction. When things go wrong with this process, it is understandable that anxiety levels in parents, not to mention professionals, become raised. Consequently, there are inevitable difficulties not only for the child but also for the parents and often for the whole family.

This book is about the different approaches to feeding problems and the different applications of some of the theoretical perspectives. As its starting point, it underlines the perception of feeding problems as distinct from eating disorders. Eating disorders tend to be rare in early childhood (Lask and Bryant-Waugh 1996). The eating distress is generally accepted as being a manifestation of quite complex underlying difficulties around self-concept. Furthermore eating disorders have the core characteristics of distorted body image and fear of fatness which are markedly absent where feeding problems are concerned. Feeding problems are characterised by an inability or refusal to eat certain foods due to physiological and/ or psychosocial factors (Babbit *et al.* 1994). Currently, there is no evidence of a causative relationship between childhood feeding problems and eating disorders (Cooper and Stein 1992). Additionally, and perhaps most importantly, the term 'feeding' implies a relationship – there is one who feeds and one who is fed. This understanding is reflected in the emphasis on the feeding *process* and the link between parents and child in defining feeding problems (Lindberg *et al.* 1991). It could be argued that this emphasis is also incongruent with the notion of 'disorder': once the process of feeding becomes the focus, it makes little sense to apply the term 'feeding disorder' to a child who is only part of the equation.

While eating disorders are relatively rare in young children, feeding problems tend to be quite common. Most children will go through periods of food refusal or faddiness and this is entirely within the range of normal behaviours during the early years. With appropriate management, these difficulties usually resolve themselves. For some children, however, this is not the case. Problems do not resolve themselves and can prove very resistant to change. In some cases, without skilled intervention they can become life-threatening. These cases may be thought of as lying further towards the 'clinical' end of the feeding problems continuum. They are usually identifiable by complex matrices of professionals and interventions. At the extreme end, children may be maintained on nasogastric tube feeding in the community for long periods, sometimes years, requiring considerable involvement of community and acute paediatrics, dietetics, community paediatric nursing, speech therapy and psychological services.

The inherently multidisciplinary nature of feeding problems means that there are typically a number of professionals involved, each focusing on a different aspect of the problem. Those involved often find themselves taking conflicting positions or representing different interests. Coupled with the very emotive nature of the problem, this adds to the overall complexity of the work. It also limits possibilities for the well-coordinated response which many see as an essential prerequisite for successful therapeutic intervention, a view echoed by current child health policy which emphasises the need for teamwork and collaboration.

Additionally, the reorientation of health services over recent years has led to an increase in focus on evidence-based medicine and measurement of therapeutic outcomes. Consequently, the cost-effectiveness of all treatment regimes is under scrutiny. This, combined with the opening up of paediatrics as a legitimate area for increased psychological as well as sociological focus, means that more and more professionals working with children and families are finding themselves called upon to help with feeding problems.

Despite the scale of the problem and the scope for useful intervention, there is remarkably little literature on the subject. Those authors who have written on the subject have tended either to equate feeding problems with eating disorders or to discuss both within the same text, which might imply a developmental continuum between the two (e.g. Cooper and Stein 1992; Lask and Bryant Waugh 1996). There have been further isolated contributions from quite disparate perspectives, but so far there has been no attempt to integrate these areas within clinical paediatrics. This book proposes to address this issue, both by exploring the interrelationship of various aspects of feeding within a multidisciplinary perspective and by focusing on clinical issues. An applied emphasis will be maintained throughout.

The chapters contained in this book concern the nature, development, maintenance and treatment of feeding problems. The text is divided into two parts: 'approaches', where the more theoretical frameworks will be discussed, and 'applications', focusing on clinical or applied research aspects of children's feeding. The initial chapter by Mary Wickendon outlines the development of oral-motor skills needed for feeding and summarises some of the ways speech and language therapists help with the acquisition of these skills. This is followed by Charles Essex's presentation of the medical approach to feeding problems through his work as a community paediatrician. Since this is the first point of contact for many children with feeding problems, as well as those who help them, this chapter provides an appropriate backdrop for exploring frontline health professional involvement further. Jo Douglas then provides an overview of psychological factors and presents a psychological framework for the assessment, classification and treatment of feeding problems based on social learning theory. The chapter by Stephen Briggs concerns the psychodyamic aspects of feeding and has a particular focus on the mother–infant relationship. Gillian Harris examines the psychophysiological and regulatory mechanisms in the aetiology of feeding. She presents an interactional model, in which the cognitive aspects and developmental characteristics of the child are examined. There follows a discussion by Kedar Dwivedi of underlying cultural aspects and beliefs as they relate to food and feeding. The 'approaches' section concludes with Angela Southall's synthesis of various aspects of feeding by highlighting the importance of the systemic dimension with her chapter on the family and wider system. The overarching aim of the editors in presenting these 'core' areas is to give the reader 'food for thought' with which to approach and inform the reading of Part 2: 'Applications', which looks at some of the ways in which these different but complementary approaches are applied.

The 'applications' part of the book outlines a number of salient, applied clinical and research areas. Some of these chapters 'map' on to those in the 'approaches' section. For example, the chapter by Mary Smale on breast-feeding makes interesting reading following Stephen Briggs's earlier discussion of psychodynamic aspects of feeding. Similarly, Jo Douglas's second chapter on selective eating builds on her earlier chapter concerning behavioural approaches to assessment and treatment. Later chapters pick up the multi-disciplinary thread, with the two chapters by Sheena Reilly, Alison Wisbeach and Lucinda Carr presenting their work on the assessment and treatment of children with neurological impairments. These chapters take an integrationist perspective, highlighting the collaborative working of speech and language therapy, occupational therapy and paediatric neurology. Specific interventions with children who are tube fed are then explored by Mandy Bryon, while the area of feeding problems in children with chronic conditions is covered by Anthony Schwartz. Following Kedar Dwivedi's earlier discussion of cultural influences on feeding, Patti Rao looks at practical issues involved in helping families whose cultural background may be different from that of their helper. Finally, the establishing and evaluation of feeding clinics are discussed by Sally Hodges and Rebecca Harris, while Jacqui Mitchell and Katie Thomas share their experiences of developing a multidisciplinary community feeding service. Hopefully, these chapters will whet the appetite of some of the readers of this book who may want to go on and do the same.

Angela Southall
Anthony Schwartz
October 1999

References

Babbit RL, Hoch TA, Coe DA *et al.* (1994) Behavioural assessment and treatment of paediatric feeding disorders. *Developmental and Behavioral Pediatrics.* **15**: 278–91.

Cooper PJ and Stein A (1992) *Feeding Problems and Eating Disorders in Children and Adolescents.* Harwood Academic Publishers, Chur, Switzerland.

Lask B and Bryant-Waugh R (1993) *Childhood Onset Anorexia Nervosa and Related Eating Disorders.* Lawrence Erlbaum Associates, Hove.

Lindberg L, Bohlin G and Hagekull B (1991) Early feeding problems in a normal population. *International Journal of Eating Disorders.* **10**: 395–405.

List of contributors

Stephen Briggs
Senior Clinical Lecturer in Social Work
Adolescent Department
The Tavistock Clinic
London

Mandy Bryon
Clinical Psychologist
Department of Psychological Medicine
The Institute of Child Health/Great Ormond Street Hospital
London

Lucinda Carr
Consultant Paediatric Neurologist
The Institute of Child Health/Great Ormond Street Hospital
London

Jo Douglas
Consultant Clinical Psychologist
Department of Psychological Medicine
The Institute of Child Health/Great Ormond Street Hospital
London

Kedar Nath Dwivedi
Consultant Child, Adolescent and Family Psychiatrist
Child and Family Consultation Service
Northampton

Charles Essex
Consultant Neurodevelopmental Paediatrician
Child Development Unit
Gulson Hospital
Coventry

Gillian Harris
Clinical Psychologist and Lecturer in Child Development
School of Psychology
University of Birmingham

Rebecca Harris
Specialist Speech and Language Therapist
Redbridge Children's Centre
London

Sally Hodges
Clinical Psychologist
Tavistock & Portman NHS Trust
London

Jacqui Mitchell
Social Worker
Child Psychiatry Department
Gulson Hospital
Coventry

Pratibha Rao
Consultant Paediatrician
Kettering General Hospital

Sheena Reilly
Professor of Speech Pathology
Royal Children's Hospital
Bundoora, Australia

Anthony Schwartz
Clinical Psychologist – Child Health
Clinical Psychology Service
The Foundation NHS Trust
Cannock

Mary Smale
Breast-feeding Counsellor and Tutor
National Childbirth Trust

Angela Southall
Consultant Clinical Psychologist – Child Health
Clinical Psychology Service
The Foundation NHS Trust
Cannock

Katie Thomas
Senior Dietician
Gulson Hospital
Coventry

Mary Wickendon
Speech and Language Therapist
Department of Human Communication
De Montfort University
Leicester

Alison Wisbeach
Head Occupational Therapist
The Institute of Child Health/Great Ormond Street Hospital
London

PART 1

APPROACHES

The development and disruption of feeding skills: how speech and language therapists can help

Mary Wickendon

Introduction

This chapter outlines the normal development of feeding skills from conception to 3 years as a foundation for looking at the ways in which this development may be disrupted. It examines a number of situations where speech and language therapy skills are brought to bear, at both the assessment and treatment stages. Detailed assessment of oral-motor and oral-sensory skills are important in gaining an overall picture of the child with feeding problems. Additionally, specific assessment of the child's communication development may reveal important factors that contribute to a wider view of the problem. Sometimes assessment of a child's oromotor skills is necessary to exclude a neurological aetiology and so enable a focus on sensory and experiential aspects of the feeding problem.

It is often difficult to isolate any specific oral problems from the perhaps much more obvious behavioural difficulties that may abound; this is when a multidisciplinary approach becomes crucial. Until quite recently, there was a tendency to categorise children with no obvious oral-motor problems as having a 'behavioural feeding problem'. This categorisation has not proved very helpful, however, as it immediately raises further questions of why these children are apparently 'anti-feeding'. The possibility of very real sensory disturbance either as a soft neurological effect or as a result of experience is now being acknowledged as contributing to children's feeding problems. The child's inability to respond normally to sensation (i.e. either over- or under-responding or both) thus needs to be considered as the possible root of the difficult behaviour, which is more obvious. This is not to say that primary psychological causes of feeding problems do not exist (and they are discussed amply elsewhere in this book), but that caution should be exercised when ruling out subtle oral-motor or oral-sensory disorders.

In order to develop a fuller sense of the importance of these factors, it is necessary to understand something of the development of the skills needed for feeding. An overview of the normal development of eating and drinking skills up to 3 years is presented. The chapter then goes on to discuss ways in which this development can be disrupted in the context of a variety of medical conditions and interventions.

Normal development of oral skills

Conception to birth

Oral activity begins very early in life, well before it is needed for feeding proper. Mouth opening in response to perioral stimulation can be seen in the fetus from around 9.5 weeks gestation, and between 10 and 17 weeks swallowing is evident. The fetus is swallowing amniotic fluid at this stage, and problems with swallowing can be indicated by polyhydramnios (excess amniotic fluid) during pregnancy. At 32 weeks a clear gag reflex is observable, quickly followed by the emergence of the cough reflex. These two reflexes are essential for airway protection immediately after birth, and throughout life.

Sucking also begins *in utero* and it is important to distinguish between two different types of suck. The non-nutritive suck is first seen in the fetus between 18 and 30 weeks. This is a fast (two per second), 'non-feeding' suck, which although rhythmical does not need to be coordinated with swallowing. Breathing after birth is through the nose, and is not interrupted by non-nutritive sucking. There is substantial evidence that this suck has comforting, settling and organising effects on the baby (Field *et al.* 1982; Measel and Anderson 1979). It is this fast, shallow action that is observable when the baby sucks their thumb *in utero* and on a dummy or other object once born. The second type of suck is the nutritive or 'active feeding' suck, which is more mature and complex and is designed to deal with fluid. It can be seen first in the 34–37-week-old, and necessitates coordination of the suck, swallow and respiration. Again it is strongly rhythmical, but is much slower (one per second) and appears more effortful. The usual pattern is for suck and swallow to be in a one-to-one relationship (i.e. suck, swallow alternating). Again breathing is nasal, and remains smooth and rhythmical, although there is a momentary pause in respiration during the swallow. The normal pattern is for a swallow always to be followed by an expiration and this makes good sense as it protects the baby's airway by expelling any material that might be in the laryngeal region threatening to be aspirated into the airway.

Sucking occurs in a 'burst–pause' pattern. Babies under 37 weeks manage 3–5 sucks in a burst and then pause for an equal interval before starting up again. They often delay swallowing and breathing until the pauses, rather than integrating them into the sucking sequence. They may therefore have periods of apnoea during feeding and may appear breathless and in need of rests. Babies over 37 weeks usually sustain nutritive sucking in bursts of 10–30 sucks and then pause for a shorter time, before another burst (more than 2 seconds between sucks counts as a pause). This is obviously more efficient as swallowing and breathing are integrated into the sequence and there is proportionately more feeding time and less resting.

Normal babies will sometimes change to non-nutritive sucking during feeding, presumably to rest. Sucking is a flexion activity, the body being curled up with the limbs held bent and in towards the body. The ideal position for efficient feeding both *in utero* and post-delivery is a flexed one. Premature babies are often unable to maintain this position and need help to stay flexed through careful handling by the carer.

Birth to three months

Efficient feeding is usually established within a few hours or days of birth in the normal term baby over 1900 grams in weight. At this stage it is a reflex-driven activity, is coordinated, smooth, rhythmical and regulated by the baby whether breast- or bottle-fed. Non-nutritive sucking can be seen at non-feeding times, particularly in the 30 minutes before a feed when the baby is hungry. The baby is able to make the transition from non-nutritive activity to a nutritive suck within a matter of seconds on receiving a nipple or teat in the mouth. The jaw and cheeks are very active in sucking and can be seen vigorously pumping up and down. The tongue makes predominantly forwards and backwards movements, with most activity in the body and back of the tongue, the tip being tucked under the teat. The tongue forms a central groove, which helps to propel the milk back towards the pharynx. The lips are open but not very active at this stage. There are two phases to the suck, expression and suction. This early sucking pattern is often referred to as 'suckling'. Both motor and sensory components are important in facilitating control of the bolus and timing the trigger of the swallow. For more detailed information about early feeding development the reader is referred to Arvedson and Brodsky (1993).

The development of these complex, coordinated skills is rapid. Physiological, neuroanatomical and psychological aspects of feeding interweave in a dynamic and fast-changing way. The more experience the baby has, the more refined and efficient the system becomes. During the first few months of life, patterns of feeding behaviour become established. A typical normal baby will manage about 113 grams of milk in 5 minutes and 227 grams in 10–15 minutes. The baby controls the speed, volume and timing of bursts and pauses during feeding. The burst–pause pattern is very obvious on observation and has been likened to early conversation, as it has a turn-taking element. Often the mother will say something to the baby during the pauses, and eye contact seems to be maintained. This is felt to be an important foundation for mother–child interaction patterns (*see* Chapter 4). The mother quickly becomes an expert at interpreting the baby's feeding activity and is able to make judgements about whether he or she is hungry, full or uncomfortable.

Three months to six months

During the second three months of life, the dynamic feeding system continues to change and develop. The baby will now be fast and efficient at sucking and will probably also be getting very good at expressing hunger, discomfort or satiation clearly. The physical position in which young babies are fed complements their anatomy at this stage. Up to about three months the proportions and arrangement of structures in the pharynx are different from those of older infants, children and adults. The small baby effectively has anatomical protection from the dangers of aspiration (penetration of food into the airways) by virtue of the position of the larynx and tongue. The larynx is much higher up in the neck, tucked under the tongue , and the epiglottis and soft palate can make contact. Thus the normal position in which to feed a young baby is a supine one. Aspiration, even in the neurologically compromised child, is unlikely. However, between three and six months this arrangement evolves so that the proportions and relationships become more like those of an older child. The chance of penetration of material into the airway is actually greater in the mature anatomy, and the position of the head becomes important, especially in the child with possible dysphagia.

As the child develops good head control and moves towards sitting balance, the mother automatically starts to adapt the feeding position to a more upright, semi-sitting one. The sucking pattern matures as the tongue begins to move up and down as well as backwards and forwards, and the lips become more active in sealing around the teat.

At some time during this stage the mother will wean the baby on to runny, puréed food from a spoon. Initially the baby takes this new food texture using old oral motor skills, i.e. s/he continues to suck. However, over a few weeks or months, many of the early feeding reflexes fade away and the child learns to have more volitional control over oral movements and develops a new range of movements, particularly of the jaw and tongue. The mother gradually expands the range of tastes and textures that the baby will accept and enjoy. The development of taste preferences is discussed elsewhere in this book (*see* Chapter 5). Different textures of food provide valuable learning opportunities for the baby, from both the sensory and motor points of view. The sensations of different textures and tastes (e.g. slimy, granular, hot, cold) stimulate the child to perceive, tolerate and habituate to a variety of foods.

The perception of the differences between textures seems to stimulate the development of a broader range of motor skills. The absence of a teat or nipple in the mouth leaves more space for tongue-tip movement. The child gradually learns to control food coming off the spoon with more discrete jaw, lip and tongue movements.

Six months to one year

During the next six months the infant become increasingly active in meal times. They will be learning early self-feeding skills, such as holding a biscuit and grabbing at the spoon. The range of tastes and textures eaten will expand greatly during this time. The child will manage to eat quite hard foods, such as breadsticks and carrots, mainly by sucking them and breaking pieces off. The child is unlikely to choke, as large lumps will easily be ejected by a strong cough and a push out by the tongue. Chewing is at a preliminary stage, effectively an up and down 'munching' movement. Many babies may be weaned on to drinking from a cup or spouted beaker at this stage, although they may continue to have breast- or bottle-feeds as well. Drinking from a cup involves abandoning sucking for more controlled lip, jaw and tongue-tip activity.

Non-feeding oral activity continues to be important and normal at this stage. Many babies enjoy non-nutritive sucking on a dummy or other favourite object and there are no reasons to discourage this at this age. Many of the early oral reflexes begin to fade out as voluntary control takes over, but spontaneous oral activity continues throughout life and performs the function of keeping the mouth clean and washed with saliva. Children learn to control saliva by closing their lips and swallowing as necessary. They may be quite dribbly at this age as they are learning to control food and saliva effectively.

Eating and drinking is a messy business, as the child wants to feel the food with his or her fingers both before and after committing it to the mouth. When eating difficult textures, many children will help themselves by moving the food around their mouth with their fingers. This is important experience, and links between manual and oral activity are regarded as part of the normal development of an integrated sensory system.

The second year

Between 12 and 24 months the toddler becomes a more skilled eater and learns to chew and bite with control. The oral and pharyngeal stages of swallowing become separable, so that the child can decide not to swallow something and can hold it tantalisingly in their mouth. The tongue develops a range of more complex movements, including tipping and side-to-side movements, and a more defined use of the tip. Children become able to eat mixed textures, which requires more sorting in the mouth of the various constituents (e.g. meat, gravy and soft vegetable in one spoonful needs skilled sorting and control by the tongue). The child may be fiercely suspicious of new experiences generally and this includes new tastes and textures. However, they enjoy exploration of new foods given an atmosphere in which they are in control.

Subsequent developments in childhood

The fine-tuning of eating and drinking skills continues over the next two years or so. The child learns to bite, chew and swallow a complete range of textures, including very chewy, very hard and mixed foods. They learn to keep their lips closed during eating, which is mainly a social convention but does cut down on spillage. The tongue is able to move accurately to retrieve food lost outside the lips or stuck around teeth and cheeks. Children also learn to tolerate and enjoy changes in tastes and learn to express their preferences verbally. Social aspects of meal times become more important as the child has increasing opportunities to eat outside his or her own home and family.

Types of feeding difficulty

Causes of feeding difficulties may be many and varied, depending on the medical and experiential history of the child. Nevertheless, the actual effects on the child's feeding behaviour can be described and categorised functionally. This is helpful, in that it leads more clearly to intervention approaches. In young babies, the distinction between 'dysfunctional' and 'disorganised' feeding is emerging as important, and in infants and older children this evolves into possible and/or sensory difficulties.

Dysfunctional versus disorganised patterns

Palmer et al. (1993a) suggested that there are two distinct and distinguishable groups of difficulty, and that it is useful to aim for a differential diagnosis between them. Palmer's work with premature and young babies suggests that those with difficulties can be grouped as either dysfunctional or disorganised (*see* Table 1.1). The NOMAS assessment records in detail the activity of the jaw, lips and tongue in both non-nutritive and nutritive sucking. She has achieved good interrater reliability judgements of these features, and the overall profile of the child across a range of features provides a picture of normal, dysfunctional or disorganised feeding. Follow-up of these children suggests that dysfunctional feeding as a baby does not resolve over time and later attracts diagnoses of neurological involvement and continued motor difficulties. Disorganised feeding either resolves to normal over time or may go on to show sensory-type feeding disorders.

Research underway suggests that this dichotomy can lead usefully to different interventions and to an indication of different prognoses (Palmer *et al.* 1993b). Thus the question 'does the child have an oral motor difficulty?' is an important one, but so also is 'does the child have oral sensory difficulty'. There may not be a diagnosis of frank cerebral palsy or other neurological disorder but more a subtle movement and coordination problem with oral movement or a disturbance of sensation.

Of course any detailed assessment of this kind is only as good as the assessor who administers it, and although Palmer achieved reliable results with her researchers, it has to be said that this is by no means an easy skill to acquire. If her link between dysfunctional features and later neurological difficulties is a true one then the responsible and reliable use of this tool will be an important addition to infant assessment and a useful way to view a complex problem. This kind of detailed oral assessment does, however, require rigorous training before it can be relied upon.

Types of intervention

Once the main processes that are maintaining the feeding problem have been identified, there are usually a number of different approaches and elements to any intervention. If the child has a mainly motor-based problem, changes to the positioning and physical support of the child will be crucial. Specific help with jaw, tongue and lip movements may be suggested. Choice of textures of food, both to prevent difficulties and encourage development of skills, will be important. There is also a balance to be struck between the nutritional needs of the child, possibly met by easy foods, and the need to challenge and stimulate new skills with more difficult foods. Taste can also play an important part in stimulating oral activity and increased movement. For more information about children with neurological involvement see Chapters 10 and 11.

Sensory problems are likely to be tackled through a combination of changes to tastes, textures and meal-time situations, the aim being to build in confidence and enjoyment of food and an expanded range of skills and experiences. The

Table 1.1: Feeding difficulties

Normal	Disorganisation	Dysfunction
Jaw		
• Consistent degree of jaw depression	• Inconsistent degree of jaw depression	• Excessively wide excursions that interrupt intra-oral seal on nipple
• Rhythmic excursions	• Arrhythmic jaw movements	• Minimal excursions; clenching
• Spontaneous jaw excursions occur on tactile presentation of nipple up to 30 minutes before a feeding	• Difficulty initiating movements: —inability to latch on —small, tremorlike start-up movements noted —does not respond to initial cue of nipple, until jiggled	• Asymmetry; lateral jaw deviation
• Jaw movement occurs at the rate of approximately 1/sec (half rate of non-nutritive suck)		• Absence of movement (% of time)
• Sufficient closure on nipple during expression phase to express fluid from nipple	• Persistence of immature suck pattern beyond appropriate age	• Lack of rate change between non-nutritive suck and nutritive suck (non-nutritive suck = 2/sec; nutritive suck = 1/sec)
Tongue		
• Cupped tongue configuration (tongue groove) maintained during sucking	• Excessive protrusion beyond labial border during extension phase of sucking without interrupting sucking rhythm	• Flaccid; flattened with absent tongue groove
• Extension-elevation-retraction movements occur in anterior-posterior direction	• Arrhythmic movements	• Retracted; humped and pulled back into oropharynx
• Rhythmic movements	• Unable to sustain suckle pattern for 2 minutes because of: —habituation —poor respiration —fatigue	• Asymmetry; lateral tongue deviation
• Movements occur at the rate of 1/sec	• Incoordination of suck or swallow and respiration, which results in nasal flaring, head turning, extraneous movement	• Excessive protrusion beyond labial border before or after nipple insertion with out and down movement
• Liquid is sucked efficiently into oropharynx for swallow		• Absence of movement (% of time)

Assessment:

Recommendations:

Therapist

timing and type of meals may be changed and there may be the addition of food-based play and more social reinforcement of positive feeding behaviours. The child may need to build up tolerance of new sensations. Often not all the changes that need to be made can be implemented at once and a planned approach is crucial. The child may need to continue to be fed on 'easy' foods for some time, with changes and variety being introduced gradually. Methods for overcoming these difficulties range in approach. Some practitioners adopt a behaviourist approach and encourage the pairing of the feeding experience with positive feedback and social reinforcement, others emphasise the need to give the child as much control and choice as possible. Some clinicians advocate sensory bombardment techniques, such as stuffing, massaging and playing around the face and mouth, to desensitise the child and normalise their response to sensations. In all cases the approach should be tailor-made for the individual, in collaboration with the parents and all the professionals involved. Advice to medical and nursing staff about reducing the aversive effects of some procedures is valuable (e.g. administering unpleasant drugs by tube, encouraging non-nutritive oral activity, encouraging the child to self-feed, the use of consistent feeders, the role of social reinforcement and interaction in feeding, the use of appropriate utensils). Often a combination of the methods mentioned above will be adopted. In all cases it is important for everyone concerned to be clear about the techniques and aims adopted and for them to be used systematically.

Motor versus sensory problems

Motor and sensory aspects obviously develop simultaneously and interact with each other in the normal development of feeding skills. However, it can be helpful to think about motor and sensory difficulties separately, although of course in many children both may be in evidence and may exacerbate each other. For instance, children who have difficulty with movements generally may have less experience of sensation because they can't get their hands to their mouths to explore at the normal stage. This may then lead to a dislike of touch around the face and mouth and refusal to try new foods, as well as poor oral movement. Conversely, children who have essentially normal motor skills but have had many aversive sensations around the mouth, such as suction, passing of tubes, or medicines, may be unwilling to try new experiences and thus do not practise new motor skills, such as coping with lumps, chewing or biting. Gisell (1991) has shown that children will use the easiest motor skills possible for any food. This suggests that if children can manage a meal by sucking (e.g. puréed vegetable and yoghurt), they will, and therefore will not be precipitated into developing more mature oral movements required by more challenging food textures. Thus there is a subtle interaction between movement and sensation, and between experience and learning new skills. It can sometimes be difficult to work out which is the primary problem, the

Table 1.2: Oral feeding disorders assessment

	Sensory	*Motor*
1 Normal oral-motor patterns	Yes	No
2 Liquids are easier to manage than textured or strained food	Yes	No
3 Mixed consistencies are difficult	No	Yes
4 Able to chew solids well	Yes	No
5 Gags when food approaches or contacts lip	Yes	No
6 Holds food to avoid swallowing	Yes	No
7 Hypersensitive gag for solids with normal liquid swallow	Yes	No

movement or the sensation. Careful analysis of the child's willingness and ability to manage different tastes and textures can often clarify this issue. Palmer and Heyman (1993) summarised this neatly, as shown in Table 1.2.

Children at risk of oral-motor or oral-sensory problems

There are a number of medical conditions that place children at risk of feeding difficulties. Of course any child may fall into more than one category, in which case their problems may be compounded and the presenting difficulty may be complex and multifactorial in aetiology. There will almost certainly be a mixture of physiological, psychological and experiential factors.

Prematurity

Premature babies do not necessarily have a problem with feeding, they are just at an earlier stage. A baby delivered at under 34 weeks will have a non-nutritive suck but is not yet neurologically ready to suck nutritively. She or he may have additional complications, such as cardiac, respiratory or gastrointestinal problems, which can affect feeding, but in the absence of these, appropriately timed introduction of oral feeding should lead to normal feeding development. The premature baby is at risk of developing sensory feeding difficulties because of the likelihood of having potentially aversive experiences, such as tube-feeding, sucking out, exhaustion, etc. Careful and sensitive management of the very young baby's feeding development is increasingly being recognised as important (Field *et al.* 1982). The provision of opportunities for non-nutritive sucking has been shown to be beneficial even when oral feeding *per se* is not yet expected. Thus a distinction in intervention can be made between oral therapy and feeding therapy, the former being appropriate when the child is not developmentally ready for the latter (Morris and Klein 1987).

Case example 1: Joshua was born at 32 weeks and weighed 1600 g, he had bronchopulmonary dysplasia. He appeared distressed and easily tired if handled but sucked well on a dummy. He was tube-fed for three weeks with use of the dummy between feeds. When started on oral feeds at 35 weeks, he took only 10 ml before tiring and appeared irritable. He took a few seconds to initiate sucking and paused after 3– 4 sucks for a rest. Over the next four weeks there was a gradual increase in the amount taken per feed. Feeding was carried out in low-stimulation surroundings and timing of pauses between bursts of sucking was structured by the feeder to allow rests and respiratory recovery. He increased his burst length to 15–20 by 38 weeks and continued to do well subsequently.

Speech and language therapy involvement in specific medical conditions

Speech and language therapists are involved in the assessment and treatment of feeding problems in children with a wide range of medical conditions. For example, in cardiac and respiratory disease, the main challenge for children is the coordination of feeding and respiration. They can easily become breathless, apnoeic and exhausted during feeding, which may compromise the whole process, and thus an efficient and effective feeding regime may not easily be established. Their feeding pattern is quite likely to fall into the disorganised category (Palmer *et al.* 1993b) and they are then at risk of disruption to sensory and psychological aspects of feeding. They need careful management of the quantity and timing of feeding so that they do not become anoxic or overtired. Their capacity to take enough feed orally may be reduced, so supplemental tube-feeding is often used. The gradual increase in oral feeding and reduction of tube-feeding requires careful staging and team discussion. Changes to feeding practice, such as maximising the positive effect of positioning, using special teats, and feeding little and often, can also contribute to success for this group.

Similarly, speech and language therapy skills may be called upon to help in the assessment and treatment of children with abnormalities of gut structure or function, such as necrotising enterocolitis, coeliac or Crohn's disease, gastroschisis, and various malabsorption and dysmotility disorders. These children are often reluctant or difficult feeders. In the absence of neurological complications they do not usually have oromotor problems but are prone to disturbances of appetite and sensation. They are a group who are likely to have had extensive medical and/or surgical intervention and prolonged hospital stays. The chances are high that experiences such as vomiting, constipation, diarrhoea, gastro-oesophageal reflux, oesophagitis, tube-feeding, medication by mouth and operative procedures will have an aversive effect on oral feeding in particular. Children may need supplemental feeding by nasogastric or gastrostomy tube or total parenteral nutrition (central line into vein). The amount, timing and type of oral feeding needs sensitive planning within the multi-professional team. It may take many months to build up the child's confidence with, and enjoyment of, eating and drinking, and it is important that the total nutritional regime for a child is planned to foster a positive attitude to oral activity and feeding as well as adequate intake (Gryboski 1975).

> *Case example 2: Catherine was a girl of 18 months with gastroschisis (malformation of the gut, with part of it outside the abdominal wall at birth). She had been in hospital and fed by a combination of nasogastric tube and central line from birth. She responded well to non-nutritive oral activities, including sucking, licking, vocalising and food-related play with dolls. She was, however, very fussy about textures, both in her mouth and on her hands. Through play she was introduced to a variety of sensations of both foods and non-foods. She showed potentially normal oromotor skills but was resistant to any foods except a bottle and puréed fruit. She was very unwilling to try a new food unless left by herself to try it. She was not able to eat more than a small quantity of food by mouth because of her gut abnormalities but therapy did result in a wider range of tastes and textures and an increased range of oromotor skills, appropriate for her age.*

Neurological disorders

Neurological disturbance, whether as a result of congenital, degenerative or acquired conditions, will clearly predispose the child to both oromotor and swallowing dysfunction (dysphagia) and to sensory abnormality (Tuchman 1989). The largest group of children presenting with neurologically based feeding difficulties are those with cerebral palsy, discussed at length in Chapters 10 and 11. It should, however, be remembered that there are more specific conditions, such as Moebius syndrome and Worster–Drought, affecting the oral musculature only. Many clinicians would agree that children with syndromes such as Retts, Williams and autism have increased incidences of feeding problems, though detailed research about these is sparse, and often it is unclear whether these have a neurological component; they may have sometimes. Some interesting work on the specific problems for children with Down's syndrome has been carried out recently by Bolders Frazier and Friedman (1996) and Spender *et al.* (1996), suggesting that their hypotonicity and hypersensitivity are likely to cause problems. Children with degenerative conditions, or who have survived anoxia or head injury, often have feeding difficulties as part of their neurological disorders. Children with less easily defined and more subtle motor dysfunction, such as those with dyspraxia and soft neurological signs, are among the most difficult to assess and define from the feeding point of view. Abnormal tone (increased, decreased or fluctuating) leads to postural problems and reduced control and muscle power for feeding. Gastro-oesophageal reflux is also a complicating factor for many children in this group and is discussed in Chapter 11. There are several good publications that cover intervention for neurologically disordered children in particular (*see* Further reading).

Developmental delay

Mild, moderate or severe developmental delay and learning difficulties are often precursors of a range of difficulties with feeding development. This may be in the absence of obvious anatomical or physiological abnormality. If cognitive, social and communication development are delayed then it is likely that feeding development will be also. Recognition that the child's feeding skills may appear poor but are actually in line with their overall development can be important in planning management and in reassuring and advising carers. Unrealistic expectations about a child's feeding skills can cause problems in themselves.

> *Case example 3: Philip was a boy with Down's syndrome referred for help with feeding at two years. He had delayed motor skills and was not yet sitting well without support. He was unable to eat any textures other than liquids and purées. More solid foods were dropped out of his mouth and his mother interpreted this as rejection. He had marked hypotonicity of his tongue, lips and jaw. Explanation that his level of oral ability was reflective of his general development and low tone was reassuring to his mother. This reduced her anxiety and helped her to understand that his apparent resistance to harder foods was probably not through dislike but because of physical difficulty and possibly some hypersensitivity. She was given advice about oral activities to increase Philip's tone and range of movements and to normalise sensation by giving him a variety of tastes and textures very regularly.*

Prolonged and complex medical intervention

Children who are very sick, have undergone major surgery or other invasive medical treatment and prolonged hospital stays are at risk of feeding problems. These can be sensory or motor in nature, quite apart from any psychological effect such experiences may have. The age at which this medical or surgical intervention has taken place is important. A child who has been in and out of hospital from infancy may never have established appropriate feeding routines and skills. The normal development of oral skills in the home environment, accompanied by social context and enjoyment, may have been disrupted. Other children may have learnt to eat normally and then developed a condition, the treatment of which exposes them to potentially aversive experiences. If the child is neurologically intact they are unlikely to have any frank oromotor problems. However, they may then appear to regress, for instance refusing all but puréed textures having previously been a competent eater of mixed foods. Children can become very fussy about both tastes and textures. This can be seen as a logical response to discomfort (such as nasogastric tube, unpleasant medicine given by mouth, frequent nausea and vomiting, intubation, etc.). Assessment of the child's oromotor skills is important in order to exclude a neurological aetiology and so focus on sensory and experiential aspects as the most likely precipitating factors. Children who are likely to fall into this group include those undergoing chemotherapy, those exposed to drugs *in utero* or later and those undergoing major surgery.

> *Case example 4: Tara was a 2:6-year-old with previously normal feeding skills, undergoing treatment for leukaemia, including chemotherapy and bone marrow transplant. While in hospital she was fed mainly by nasogastric tube to keep her weight up and although she was encouraged to eat as well, this was reduced to very occasional soft foods. She was happy to touch and explore other foods but if it were suggested that she put them in her mouth she would gag (conditioned gag). She was encouraged to feed herself and gradually gained confidence with a wide range of purées, mousses, etc. However, she did not make major improvements until she was at home and had some meals without the tube* in situ. *She quickly showed very good oromotor skills but remained fussy about new textures and mixed textures for a further year.*

Metabolic, liver and kidney diseases

There is mounting anecdotal evidence that children with various metabolic, liver and kidney diseases are at risk of poor feeding (*see* Chapter 13). They often appear to have disturbances of taste perception and appetite and these tend to be difficult to resolve. Of course this population are part of the larger group who are likely to have had multiple hospital stays, unpleasant procedures and periods of being unwell. They may have had little opportunity to establish normal feeding routines and skills. Their diet may necessarily be restricted, thus limiting chances to explore a range of foods. They can become extremely fussy about tastes and textures of food, influencing opportunities to develop mature oral and social skills at meal times. Often it appears that there is an oromotor component to the difficulty, but on closer assessment this is rarely the case. Concern about the child's weight may exacerbate anxiety around meal times and mean that eating becomes a highly stressful activity for both child and carers. Tube-feeding is often a necessary part of the intervention programme but it can also serve to prolong the disruption to normal oral feeding. The problems are often essentially sensory in nature. Quick-fix solutions to these types of difficulties are unlikely to be successful. Intervention often requires a combination of careful manipulation of the meal-time situation and its context and also a great deal of specific advice and reassurance to the carers about encouraging eating and making it a positive experience.

ENT disorders and unusual structure or function

There are a number of abnormalities of the oral, nasal and pharyngeal regions that may disrupt feeding. The most common of these are the various clefts of lip and/or palate, which as a group occur in one in 600 births. As a general rule, cleft just of the lip does not cause great problems; indeed mothers who wish to breast-feed these babies are often successful. Cleft palate occurs in various forms, ranging form submucous cleft where there is no obvious 'hole', as it is the underlying bone and muscle which has failed to fuse despite an intact mucosal layer, through unilateral cleft of the hard and/or soft palate to bilateral cleft, where the child has very little effective roof to the mouth. This lack of intact palate may affect the posture and function of the tongue and thus feeding efficiency. Without an efficient soft palate, which would normally elevate to close off the nose during sucking and swallowing, there is a tendency for food to enter the nasopharynx. Some cleft babies learn to direct milk posteriorly with relatively little leakage into the nose. Others are troubled by a very inefficient suck and marked nasal regurgitation, particularly of liquids. In the absence of any neurological problems, the muscle power and control of cleft babies is normal, but because of the lack of velopharyngeal closure they have difficulty building up pressure in the mouth. This results in a weak suck and often also the swallowing of air. Babies with clefts may therefore have discomfort from wind, sneezing, very long feed times and a general disinclination to feed. In the early days, much can be done to help by using specialist teats, cup and spoon feeding, and careful positioning. Once the cleft lip and/or palate have been repaired, an improvement in feeding skills can usually be expected. But this may not be immediate as the effect of negative learning about feeding, alongside the physical difficulties, may have taken its toll. Children with cranial facial syndromes, such as Crouzons, are likely to have complex feeding problems because of the combination of clefting, airway and other difficulties (for further information refer to Bannister 1999).

Much less common are the various pharyngeal and laryngeal malformations that are usually of congenital aetiology but can also arise through trauma. Laryngomalacia (literally malformed larynx) causes problems because the baby has a compromised airway. This will inevitably affect feeding, particularly if the child has a tracheostomy fitted in order to ensure an adequate airway. Children with compromised airways often adopt a characteristic extended neck position and this is an exception to the general rule that the best head position for swallowing is one where the chin is at 90 degrees to the neck. Many tracheostomised children will be neurologically intact and can quite safely swallow with an extended head. However, it is important that the efficiency of the swallow is assessed. If it is not safe they may need to be fed by tube for some time. In older children the presence of the tracheostomy may result in 'tethering' of the larynx, preventing it from elevating normally during swallowing. A marked improvement in swallowing may therefore be seen once the trachae tube is removed. A videofluoroscopic view of the oral and pharyngeal mechanisms during feeding can be very useful in these cases (Griggs *et al.* 1989). The child may be able to swallow some textures easily but have difficulty controlling liquids safely.

> *Case example 5: Bhupinder was referred at 10 months with con-genital laryngomalacia. He had had a tracheostomy in place since birth and had undergone two operations to try to remodel his larynx to ensure a safe airway. He was tube-fed until six months and then intermittently whenever he had a chest infection. He tended to be congested and short of breath and needed frequent sucking out, which his mother was able to do at home. He had normal oromotor skills and could drink well from a bottle for short periods before becoming tired and breathless. He tended to adopt an extended head position but had a safe swallow. He was interested in solid food but was tentative about new foods., Once he had tasted them he usually indicated that he wanted more. He needed to be sucked out during meals as he produced lots of mucus during oral activity and then became breathless. He enjoyed munching on breadsticks and other finger food. His mother was encouraged to feed him little and often and offer a wide variety of different textures and tastes. He showed slow but steady improvement over the following 18 months and once his trachae was removed at the age of 2:10, showed increased willingness to experiment with a variety of food types.*

Children with various types of tracheo-oesophageal fistula (TOF) also have difficulties, usually with swallowing rather than oral skills. These children have a malformation of the trachea and/or the oesophagus such that there may be a danger of food entering the trachea. This malformation is identified within the first few hours or days of life, and the child will probably then be fed by tube for some months or occasionally years. After surgical repair of the anatomy the child has gradually to be weaned on to oral feeding, and has to get used to the associated sensations both in the mouth and in the thorax and abdomen. Some hospitals advocate 'sham feeding', which is the use of oral feeding to provide practice at eating, but with the food re-routed out through a stoma in the neck rather than going into the oesophagus and gut. Thus the child is experiencing at least some aspects of oral feeding, while awaiting surgery or healing of the repair. Some TOF children continue to be reluctant feeders for many years and some are bothered by recurrent strictures around the repair site, which cause discomfort and discourage the child from eating lumpy foods. Strictures can be dilated surgically but in the meantime some adverse learning about eating may have taken place. Similar types of problems sometimes occur in children who have acquired damage to the larynx, pharynx or oesophagus through swallowing acid, physical trauma or similar accidents.

The effects of early experiences on feeding skills

Any aversive experiences which involve the oral structures or the feeding situation may affect feeding skills subsequently. These include aspiration, gastro-oesophageal reflux, oral medication, intubation, tube-feeding, breathlessness, sucking out, ventilation, force-feeding, etc. If early experiences of eating and drinking have been traumatic or difficult and have involved physical discomfort, such as coughing, choking, or pharyngeal irritation, then the likelihood of feeling positive about meal times is reduced. A child who aspirates on liquids will associate drinking with the discomfort and panic involved rather than the pleasure of the drink. Feelings of breathlessness and exhaustion during feeding will also disincline the child to persevere even if they enjoy the taste of the food. There is little clear research on the physical effects of nasogastric tubes on the functioning of the oral and pharyngeal structures. However, it seems clear clinically that some children are much more irritated by the tube than others. Many children revert to easier textures and a restricted range of tastes when they are being tube and orally fed simultaneously. Adults who have been fed by tube report discomfort and irritation that they say affects their willingness and enjoyment of eating and drinking considerably. Children who have experienced regular medical procedures involving their mouth, such as passing of tubes, ventilation or taking unpleasant medicine, may develop abnormal sensory responses to any kind of activity in the oral and facial area. This often presents in the form of fussiness about taste and texture of food or more extreme refusal. In addition to the actual negative response to the food, it should be remembered that for many children there is also the simple matter of lack of practice. If they have had problems from infancy they may never have built up the routine and skills needed to be consistently good feeders.

Tube-feeding

Anecdotally, there is evidence that nasogastric tubes affect oral feeding skills. Apart from the complex issues of appetite, parental anxiety, nutritional status, etc., which are covered elsewhere in this book, the actual mechanical feeding skills and sensations of eating do often seem to be affected by the presence of the tube. This makes intuitive sense. It has been noted that children being fed by nasogastric tube, for whatever reason, are often unwilling to eat orally (Wickendon 1992). More specifically they tend not to want to try new or lumpy textures. In some cases these are textures that they have managed well before; *see* case example 4. These children are often very good at 'training' their carers to give them only textures they can swallow comfortably with the tube in position. An improvement in their oral skills sometimes occurs soon after the tube is removed. In other cases the damage is slower in resolving. Some children appear to habituate to the sensation of the tube within a few days, others continue to sneeze, cough, pull it out or refuse to eat over prolonged periods. It has been suggested that habituating to the presence of a foreign body in the nasopharynx, although convenient initially, has disadvantages. Some children seem to become hyposensitive to stimulation in the pharynx as a result and thus do not control the bolus effectively and the pharynx becomes a desensitised 'black hole'. This has its own dangers. Although little systematic research has been carried out, many clinicians would feel that long-term nasogastric feeding is likely to have a negative effect on both the sensory and motor components of oral feeding development. These can only compound other psychological processes that may be in action. Trying to improve oral feeding in a child who is also being fed by nasogastric tube can be a frustrating and thankless task because one cannot assume a normally functioning oral system even in the absence of gross oromotor disorder. Most would welcome the more frequent use of gastrostomy feeding for children who need long-term nutritional support in addition to any oral feeding they can manage.

Interaction between different types of feeding problems

Of course there can be coexistence of several types of feeding problem. In fact it is likely that several important factors will combine to create a marked difficulty rather than there being a single cause. Sometimes it is difficult to be sure where the boundaries between, say, a motor and sensory problem or a sensory and a behavioural difficulty lie. In a sense it is an artificial boundary of only academic interest. The question of cause or effect of a resulting problem looms often and is frequently intractable in practical terms. For instance, most children who have experienced tube-feeding probably have some elements of both sensory and motor difficulty. Recognition that problems are often multi-factorial is important when planning intervention.

Summary

Normal feeding development begins *in utero* and is a dynamic physiological as well as psychological process. Progression through the stages of sucking and weaning on to more mature eating and drinking is usually smooth and unproblematic. Both the motor and sensory components of this development are important. The integration of movement and sensation with experience can easily be disrupted by a number of disease processes and/or the intervention which follows them. The reasons for feeding problems can be many and varied if a child has had a significant medical condition in infancy or childhood. In some ways it is surprising that so many children who have aversive experiences early in life eat and drink well. Progress has been made in recent years with the recognition of the existence of subtle oral-motor and oral-sensory difficulties, which can have a major effect on feeding behaviour. Some of these effects may be preventable as there is some evidence that early aversive experiences and subtle oral-motor difficulties can have significant effects on later skills and attitudes at meal times. More research is needed into the most beneficial early preventative interventions to minimise the chances of long-term feeding difficulties in children with complex medical conditions. It is clear that careful assessment of children's oral-sensory and oral-motor skills and experiences, and specific intervention advice, form an important part of the bigger picture.

References

Arvedson JC and Brodsky L (eds) (1993) *Paediatric Swallowing and Feeding: assessment and management*. Whurr, London.

Bannister P (1999) Early feeding management. In: Watson, Grunwell and Sell (eds) *Management of Cleft Lip and Palate*. Whurr, London.

Bolders Frazier J and Friedman B (1996) Swallow function in children with Down syndrome: a retrospective study. *Developmental Medicine and Child Neurology*. **38**: 695–703.

Field T, Ignatoff E, Stringer S *et al.* (1982) Non-nutritive sucking during tube feedings: effects on preterm neonates in an intensive care unit. *Paediatrics*. **70**: 381–4.

Gisell EG (1991) Effect of food texture on the development of chewing of children between six months and two years of age. *Developmental Medicine and Child Neurology*. **33**: 69–79.

Griggs CA, Jones PM and Lee RE (1989) Videofluroroscopic investigation of feeding disorders of children with multiple handicap. *Developmental Medicine and Child Neurology*. **31**: 303–8.

Gryboski J (1975) Gastrointestinal problems in the infant. In: *Major Problems in Clinical Pediatrics*. Saunders, Philadelphia, PA.

Measel CP and Anderson GC (1979) Nonnutritive sucking during tube feedings: effect on clinical course in premature infants. *Journal of Obstetric, Gynecologic and Neonatal Nursing*. **8**: 265–72.

Morris SE and Klein MD (1987) *Pre-feeding Skills: a comprehensive resource for feeding development*. Therapy Skill Builders, Tucson, AZ (available from Winslow Press, Buckingham).

Palmer MM and Heyman MB (1993) Assessment and treatment of sensory-versus motor based feeding problems in very young children. *Infants and Young Children*. **6**(2): 67–73.

Palmer MM, Crawley K and Blanco I (1993a) NOMAS: nutritive suck: tongue. *Journal of Perinatology*. **xiii**(i):30.

Palmer MM, Crawley K and Blanco I (1993b) The Neonatal Oral-Motor Assessment Scale: a reliability study. *Journal of Perinatology*. **13**: 28–35.

Spender Q, Stein A, Dennis J *et al.* (1996) An exploration of feeding difficulties in children with Down syndrome. *Developmental Medicine and Child Neurology*. **38**: 681–94.

Tuchman DN (1989) Cough, choke, splutter: the evaluation of the child with dysfunctional swallowing. *Dysphagia*. **3**: 3.

Wickendon JM (1992) Oral skills in nasogastrically fed children under 3. MSc. thesis, City University, London.

Further reading

Braun MA and Palmer MM (1985) A pilot study of oral-motor dysfunction in 'at-risk' infants. *Physical and Occupational Therapy in Pediatrics*. **5**(4): 13–25.

Bosma JF (1986) Development of feeding. *Clinical Nutrition*. **5**: 210–18.

Bu'Lock F, Woolridge MW and Baum JD (1990) Development of co-ordination of sucking, swallowing and breathing: ultrasound study of term and preterm infants. *Developmental Medicine and Child Neurology*. **32**: 669–78.

Caeser P, Daniels H, Devleiger H *et al.* (1982) Feeding behaviour in preterm neonates. *Early Human Development*. **7**: 331–46.

Kramer SS (1985) Radiological examination of the swallowing impaired child. *Dysphagia*. **3**: 117–25.

Mathisen B, Skuse D, Wolke D and Reilly S (1989) Oral-motor dysfunction and failure to thrive among inner-city infants. *Developmental Medicine and Child Neurology*. **31**: 293–302.

Morris SE (1982) *Pre-speech Assessment Scale.* J.A. Preston Corporation, New Jersey.

Morris SE (1989) Development of oral-motor skills in the neurologically impaired child receiving non-oral feedings. *Dysphagia*. **3**: 135–54.

Reilly S, Skuse D, Mathisen B and Wolke D (1995) The objective ratings of oral-motor functions during feeding. *Dysphagia*. **10**: 177–91.

Skuse D, Stevenson J, Reilly S and Mathisen B (1995) Schedule for Oral Motor Assessment (SOMA) methods of validation. *Dysphagia*. **10**: 192–202.

Vanden Berg KA (1990) Nippling management of the sick neonate in the NICU: the disorganised feeder. *Neonatal Network*. **9**(1): 9–16.

Warner J (1981) *Helping the Handicapped Child with Early Feeding*. Winslow Press, Buckingham.

Winstock A (1994) *The Practical Management of Eating and Drinking Difficulties in Children*. Winslow Press, Buckingham.

Wolf S and Glass R (1992) *Feeding and Swallowing Disorders in Infancy*. Therapy Skill Builders, Tucson, AZ.

Wolff PH (1968) The serial organisation of sucking in the young infant. *Pediatrics*. **42**(6): 943–56.

CHAPTER 2

Children with feeding difficulties: medical perspectives

Charles Essex

Introduction

As a medical doctor, a community paediatrician is trained in paediatrics, with a special emphasis on children's development. He or she is ideally placed to draw together information about the child when there is a complex difficulty or one which involves a number of professionals. Medical doctors are trained in making diagnoses, which may involve appropriate investigations and prescribing certain types of treatment. This is sometimes pejoratively called the 'medical model' (Bax 1998). However, such a focus does not exclude an awareness of the social context and environment of the child. Indeed, the community paediatrician is often in the best position to take a holistic view of the child, including the family, educational and developmental progress, in consultation with other professionals in health, education and social services, as appropriate. This chapter reviews the assessment, treatment and coordinating role of the community paediatrician in children with feeding difficulties.

Assessment

When faced with a child with possible feeding problems, it is essential for the paediatrician to take a careful history, ideally from those who have most experience of dealing with the child. This will include details around the present problem as well as other information that may be relevant. This will help to establish perceptions of the onset of the problem, how it has changed, what measures have been tried so far and with what degree of success, if any. Listening and observing how the carers describe the problem can also give valuable information, depending on the body language, tone of voice, vocabulary and mood of the speaker.

Other details can also be helpful in building up a picture of the child's background and any contributing factors. This includes details of the pregnancy, such as any health problems or drugs taken (including prescribed, over-the-counter and illicit drugs), and length of gestation, which will indicate any prematurity. By implication, if a baby is born preterm there must have been a problem, either for the baby, the mother or both. Thus the mother went into premature labour spontaneously or was induced by her obstetric attendants for her and/or the baby's well being, such as severe pregnancy-induced hypertension or fetal distress.

Details of the events surrounding the birth, such as premature rupture of membranes, the method of delivery of the baby and birth weight, can be very helpful. The method of delivery can indicate whether the baby was having problems prior to birth. For example, a caesarean section is not in itself a problem, but the reason why the baby was delivered by caesarean section may be significant. The condition of the baby immediately after birth and his or her weight are important. If a baby is small for its gestational age there may have been intrauterine growth retardation.

The Apgar score is frequently quoted (Apgar 1953). This is a practical and quick method of systematically assessing the infant immediately after birth. The Apgar score evaluates five signs (Table 2.1) at one minute and five minutes. Each sign is given a score of 0, 1 or 2. Only the first of these five signs is objective, but the Apgar score does ensure that newborn babies are observed and assessed.

The progress of the baby in the first few days post-natally can give valuable information. For example, a baby who has been taken home within a couple of days of birth has clearly not had significant perinatal problems. Conversely, babies who suffer from severe birth asphyxia or significant intracranial

Table 2.1: Apgar score

Score	0	1	2
Heart rate	absent	<100/min	>100/min
Respiratory effort	nil	slow, irregular	regular with cry
Muscle tone	limp	some tone in limbs	active moments
Reflex irritability	nil	grimace only	cry
Colour	pallor or cyanosis	body pink, extremities blue	pink all over

haemorrhage can have a very stormy time in the post-natal period, during which time they may have seizures and require ventilation and/or prolonged nasogastric feeding. A baby who has birth asphyxia sufficient to cause brain damage is almost always extremely ill with hypoxic ischaemic encephalopathy; he or she requires neonatal intensive care, ventilation and non-oral feeding, and has seizures. A baby whose oesophagus did not form properly (oesophageal atresia) did not have a functioning oesophagus *in utero* and therefore is likely to have feeding problems

Details of the child's past medical history, since the neonatal period, may reveal the need for hospital admissions or surgery. Information about the child's developmental progress will help to indicate whether developmental milestones have been reached within the appropriate time frame. Infants may be described by health professionals or parents as being 'slow' or 'late' to reach a milestone, such as walking. However, this is often in comparison to the 'average' age at which children reach that milestone. By definition, if that is the mean average, then 50% of children will have achieved that particular milestone, but 50% will not.

A family history extending beyond the members of the immediate family can be informative, as it may show that other members of the family had eating difficulties or were simply 'picky eaters'. Alternatively it may reveal serious conditions in other members of the family or numerous miscarriages, stillbirths or early infant deaths, which may indicate an underlying genetic problem. In some cases, for example where families have a particular cultural background which permits intra-familial marriage, parents should be asked specifically whether they are 'blood relatives' as consanguinity increases the risk of children having genetic disorders.

The past medical history will indicate whether the child has had any significant illnesses or operations, or other admissions to hospital requiring interventions or investigations. Parents need to be specifically asked about whether the child has ever had a nasogastric tube inserted. Details of the early feeding history, whether the child was breast- or formula-fed, feeding behaviour (including how well the child sucked), at what age breast-feeding was stopped and why, the age of introduction of solids and the progress from first baby foods, and a dietary history of the types and textures of foods the child now eats.

The child needs a thorough physical examination. This will include looking at the overall appearance of the child including any unusual facial features (called dysmorphic features), which may be characteristic of a particular syndrome, or alternatively may alert the paediatrician to a possible underlying chromosomal abnormality or undefined non-specific congenital abnormality. The skin should be looked at for any birth marks or unusual patterns of hyper- or hypopigmentation, as well as the hair (its structure and patterns of growth) (Smith and Gong 1973) and teeth. The child's height, weight and head circumference should be measured and compared to any previous measurements, if available, to get an estimate of the rate of growth. As well as a general physical examination of the child, muscle bulk should be assessed as an indication of possible malnutrition or wasting.

A careful neurological examination of muscle tone and strength, reflexes and any tremor should be done. The child should be observed walking, if appropriate, as this may reveal abnormalities such as mild cerebral palsy, which may otherwise not have been picked up. Drooling at an inappropriate age may indicate poor swallowing or poor control of muscles of the lips and mouth or neck. Abnormal eye movements, either as a squint or uncoordinated roving eye movements (nystagmus), may indicate an underlying neurological disorder.

The paediatrician can also gain much information from observing the child play, and from his or her interaction with parents and strangers such as the doctor. The child's gestures, behaviour with adults and general interest in surroundings help the paediatrician to build up an informal picture of the child's developmental abilities and developmental level.

It can be very helpful to observe how the child handles objects, whether he or she puts them to his or her mouth or not, if this is an appropriate developmental stage, or if an older child plays with toys in an imaginative way. It can be helpful to watch the child feed, which may be either breast-feeding, or drinking from a bottle or cup. (Chapter 8 outlines issues regarding breast-feeding.) Similarly, if the child is given solids such as biscuits or crisps this will also provide useful information both in terms of how they are offered to the child as well as how they are received. Careful observation must take account of evidence of any neurological problems or indications of learning disabilities, or any impairment of social, communication or imaginative play skills and repetitive non-constructive actions, which might suggest a disorder along the autistic spectrum.

Blood and urine tests may be arranged, as well as imaging techniques such as scans, although frequently these are done to exclude conditions rather than to confirm that a specific condition exists. Investigations in both neuro-developmental delay and failure to thrive are frequently unrewarding (Newton and Wraith 1995; Berwick *et al.* 1982).

Growth charts

Growth charts, also known as centile charts, are often used by both health professionals and parents as an indicator of a child's nutritional status and general well being. However, it is important that they are used appropriately and their limitations are recognised. Growth charts are compiled from serial measurements of a group of children, who are presumed to be normal, over a period of time. Growth charts most commonly used are those for weight, height and head circumference, although centile charts are available for chest circumference, hand measurements, foot length, eye measurements, ear length, penile and testicular growth. Growth charts are also available for children with some syndromes, including Down's syndrome, Cornelia de Lange syndrome and Turner's syndrome.

Traditionally the growth charts have been drawn with the 97th, 90th, 75th, 50th, 25th, 10th and 3rd centiles. Recently growth charts have been produced which range from the 99.6th centile to the 0.4 centile. However, to get the maximum benefit from growth charts, measurements must be made correctly, plotted correctly and interpreted correctly. It is important to take into account familial growth patterns. Short parents tend to produce short children and vice versa; a significant number of children seen in growth clinics because of short stature are only following their familial trend (*see* Chapter 5).

It is generally accepted that allowance must be made for prematurity when plotting measurements on the growth chart. In other words, if the child was born, say, eight weeks prematurely, then eight weeks should be deducted from the child's chronological age. What is less clear is how long this allowance for prematurity should be made. The author continues to allow for prematurity for the duration of the first growth chart (for example, 0–2 years of age). If prematurity is ignored at some stage during the duration of a particular growth chart, for example at the child's first birthday, then a measurement at approximately 12 months would be plotted and interpreted as if the child were 10 months old. The measurement taken the next day would be virtually the same and would be plotted at 12 months of age (the child's chronological age). It would appear as if the child had had a period of arrested growth.

Developmental assessment

Children with feeding difficulties need a careful developmental assessment. This may be one of the first indicators that the child has a serious underlying problem. It will also give an indication of the child's feeding abilities, particularly the ability to communicate needs, wishes and preferences, and the ability to self-feed.

The form of multidisciplinary developmental assessment a child receives varies widely, as there have been no randomised controlled trials of the best way of performing these assessments, or even whether they are effective.

In some districts, any child referred to the local Child Developmental Centre (CDC) because of suspected developmental delay is automatically accepted for assessment. The child may be seen over a consecutive number of days by a variety of therapists and health professionals, including the speech and language therapist, occupational therapist and physiotherapist. A number of further investigations may be made, such as hearing, vision, play and dental assessments, as well as a medical examination. Sometimes both an educational psychologist and a social worker are involved. In other districts, the child may be seen for a half-day assessment weekly for a number of weeks. Some districts do not have a CDC and the child will be seen by the appropriate professionals either at home, at the local clinic or in the child's nursery setting.

In other districts, such as where the author works, the community paediatrician undertakes an initial developmental assessment. If the child shows a developmental delay affecting one or possibly two areas of development then referrals can be made to the appropriate therapists (for example, for speech therapy and for a hearing test). However, if the child is showing delay in more than two areas of development, then a multidisciplinary assessment is undertaken at the CDC.

From this, a comprehensive assessment of the child's abilities can be made and appropriate services put in place or recommendations made. This may include physical therapies, such as physiotherapy or speech therapy, psychological therapies for the child and family, educational services, such as special nursery placements, and the involvement of the educational psychologist.

Genetics

A number of conditions in which feeding difficulties may be one component have a genetic basis. A careful family history may reveal that other members of the family have had similar problems. However, recessive conditions, which require both parents to carry the responsible gene, may go undetected for several generations in a family until someone marries another unsuspecting carrier. Alternatively the child with the condition may have a new mutation: in other words, he or she may be the first person in that family to have developed an inheritable condition and is thus at risk of passing on the condition to his or her children. Chapter 13 outlines issues regarding feeding in children with chronic, inherited conditions, such as cystic fibrosis.

Genetic counselling may be done by the community paediatrician or the family can be referred to a geneticist. The family can be given an estimated risk of any future children having a similar condition. At the same time they may also be given information about the likelihood of the affected child's offspring having a similar condition. If the condition can be recognised as a syndrome (that is, a collection of symptoms and signs which constitute a known disorder) then some idea of the prognosis and likely development for the child can be given.

Treatment

If the child has a feeding problem, the fundamental aim of treatment is to ensure that sufficient calories are consumed for energy requirement and growth. Depending on the complexity of the feeding difficulty, a number of other professionals may be involved. The dietician is frequently involved in providing dietary advice and information about the use of high-calorie feeds and thickeners. His or her input is essential where any proposed changes to a feeding regime are required. Similarly, behavioural management advice may be important in order to promote changes in feeding behaviour (*see* Chapter 2).

Practical measures such as positioning may be helpful; for example in young infants with severe gastro-oesophageal reflux (GOR), placing the infant in a 30 degrees reclined sitting position will help (Larnert and Ekberg 1995).

Drug treatment

Many children who have GOR or repeated vomiting are often tried on alginate combinations (e.g. Gaviscon). These work by forming a viscous layer on top of the gastric contents. Thus if the child refluxes or vomits, the surface layer, which also contains antacids, will offer some protection to the oesophageal mucosa. The adult formulation of Gaviscon contains relatively high amounts of sodium and therefore Infant Gaviscon should be used in children under two years of age.

Prokinetic drugs are useful in that they have an effect throughout the gastrointestinal tract. These increase tightening of the oesophageal sphincter and promote gastric emptying. Cisapride is the most commonly used prokinetic drug. It can cause colic and diarrhoea, although as children with feeding difficulties often have severe neurological impairment and also constipation, the effect on the bowels may be welcome.

Drugs to reduce gastric acid secretion are used in more severe cases. These include H_2 antagonists such as cimetidine. Gastric acid secretion can also be reduced by drugs such as omeprazole, which is a proton pump inhibitor that blocks the final step in the pathway of gastric acid production.

Many children whose feeding problems are related to severe neurological impairment or to significant neurological immaturity have significant drooling. Although this is not usually distressing for the child, it can be embarrassing for parents and siblings and can also create a lot of washing for the parents as the child may require a change of clothes several times a day. Hyoscine patches can be very effective at reducing drooling. These are slow-release patches that are stuck on the skin, rather like plasters. They are impregnated with hyoscine, which is then absorbed transdermally, and are effective for up to three days.

Other more invasive treatments are sometimes used. The most frequent is a nasogastric tube. These can be used either on an intermittent basis or inserted and removed on a daily basis. They may also be left *in situ* long term.

Surgical and invasive treatments

Nasogastric tubes

Although nasogastric tubes are normally a hospital-based intervention, they are sometimes used in the community. Briefly, the advantages of nasogastric tubes are as follows:

- they can be inserted rapidly
- parents can be taught to insert them
- they allow food and medicines to be given directly into the stomach
- they can be removed easily and quickly.

Nasogastric tubes also have disadvantages. These are summarised as follows:

- frequent development of sensitivity around the mouth and nasopharynx. This can be a particular problem for children who are taking some food or drink by mouth; this oral feeding, however limited, may be lost if the child becomes sensitive or develops an aversion to things in or around his or her mouth
- the discomfort of having a foreign body in place; increased saliva production; the visual impact of the nasogastric tube if it is left in place and strapped to the face
- skin reactions from the strapping and soreness to the nose
- they do not prevent GOR.

Gastrostomy

Gastrostomies are being used increasingly for children who have prolonged periods of significant feeding difficulties in preference to continued or prolonged nasogastric feeding. In consultation with both the parents and other health professionals caring for the child, the child may be referred to a paediatric surgeon for insertion of a gastrostomy. The indications for gastrostomy are given in Box 2.1.

Gastrostomies have several advantages. These include improved nutritional access; improved growth; reduced feeding times; reduced feeding-related choking; and reduced incidence of chest infections (Elthami and Sullivan 1997; Tawfik *et al.* 1997).

However, gastrostomies also have disadvantages, both physical and psychological. The physical disadvantages include early complications, such as bleed-

> **Box 2.1:** Indications for gastrostomy
>
> Severe oral and/or pharyngeal dysphagia
> Unsafe oral feeding
> Prolonged oral feeding times
> Inadequate oral intake
> Failed oral supplementation
> Chronic food refusal
> Prolonged nasogastric tube feeding
> Increased energy needs

ing from the site of the wound, wound infections, abdominal distension, vomiting and gastroenteritis. Late complications include vomiting, retching, granulation around the wound, late infection, GOR (which can be particularly severe) and 'dumping'. 'Dumping' takes place when there is distortion of the anatomy of the stomach and interference of the normal peristaltic movements of the stomach musculature. A bolus of semi-digested food can be 'dumped' in the upper part of the small intestine and lead to abdominal discomfort, with sweating and pallor.

The disadvantages of gastrostomy feeding also include the surgical nature of the insertion of the tube, the anaesthetic and the fact that it is an 'unnatural' method of feeding – the inability of the parents to provide for the child's nutritional needs in a 'normal' way.

Children must be carefully selected for gastrostomy. This includes careful assessment of the child's nutritional needs and whether or not these are being met by other means; the views of the family on having a gastrostomy inserted; the presence of any GOR. If the child has GOR this is almost always made worse by the insertion of a gastrostomy. Children will therefore need specialised barium X-rays of the oesophagus and stomach prior to surgery.

Most paediatric surgeons would correct any GOR or perform a fundoplication (an operation in which part of the stomach is wrapped around the lower end of the oesophagus) to prevent any subsequent GOR (Heine *et al.* 1995).

Many children with feeding difficulties also have bowel problems, of which constipation is by far the most common. It is outside the remit of this chapter to discuss this issue, although a comprehensive review can be found elsewhere (Clayden 1992).

Excessive drooling

Many children with feeding problems also have problems with drooling. There are a variety of reasons for this, such as difficulty with swallowing, oromotor difficulties or nasogastric feeding. Advice on treatment for drooling should be readily available. Whereas some parents and children may not find this a problem, others will. If required, the community paediatrician can make a referral to the oral surgeon who can perform a relocation of the salivary glands as necessary, which can direct the flow of saliva backwards into the pharynx. Alternatively, the community paediatrician can prescribe hyoscine patches to help to dry up oral secretions, as described above.

Psychological treatments

There may be psychological issues for both the parents and child which relate to the child's feeding. Many parents feel guilty, upset and frustrated at a perceived inability to feed their child. There may be frequent tensions between the child and family around feeding. These psychological issues are dealt with more fully in Chapters 7 and 9.

Liaison with other health professionals

Referrals received

A community paediatrician will receive referrals from primary care workers such as GPs and health visitors because of concern about either a child's overall development or specific aspects of the child's development, in this case related to his or her feeding difficulties. Alternatively, referrals may be made by, for example, a speech therapist or physiotherapist who has seen the child at the request of a primary care worker because of perceived difficulties with speech and language or gross motor skills. The therapist will then refer to the community paediatrician for further assessment if it is felt that the child has significant difficulties and/or to exclude a more serious underlying condition.

With the increasing complexity of paediatric medicine and surgery, and the necessity to specialise, other paediatricians and paediatric surgeons will refer children with feeding problems to the community paediatrician who takes a lead role in this area.

Referrals sent

Having seen the child, the paediatrician will review the information from his or her own history and examination of the child, together with any information received from others involved with the child, including the person making the referrals. Medical knowledge and technology has expanded to such an extent that no health professional, either medical or non-medical, can maintain a working knowledge of all the pathology, investigations and treatment beyond his or her immediate field of interest or expertise. In some districts, groups of relevant professionals are forming – either formally or informally – a feeding 'team' to look at the needs of the child with feeding difficulties. Thus while the community paediatrician maintains the overall responsibility for the coordination of the child's care, he or she may often need to refer the child to other specialists, both medical and non-medical, for further investigation, diagnosis and treatment, as shown in Box 2.2.

Box 2.2: Professionals who might see a child with feeding difficulties

- Paediatric gastroenterologist: paediatrician with expertise in disorders of the gastrointestinal system
- Paediatric endocrinologist: paediatrician with expertise in disorders of the glands
- Maxillofacial, craniofacial or plastic surgeon: surgeon with expertise in operating in the area of the head and neck
- Geneticist: doctor specialising in inherited or congenital disorders
- Physiotherapist: examines physical performance, gross motor skills and body organisation
- Occupational therapist: deals with fine motor skills, hand function, activities of daily living, perception and graphic skills
- Speech therapist: specialises in the development of a child's communication skills and examines issues relating to oral and pharyngeal functioning
- Clinical psychologist: specialises in issues relating to functioning in the areas of emotional, behavioural and social development at both individual family and group levels
- Educational psychologist: psychologist with expertise in the educational needs of children with chronic or severe disorders which may interfere with access to the National Curriculum in the normal way

---

Liaison with education services

Most children with feeding problems are identified in the pre-school years. However, if the feeding difficulty is part of a wider developmental, learning or medical problem, then the child will have needs and difficulties which will probably impinge on his or her ability to access the National Curriculum in the usual way.

The special needs department of the local education authority therefore needs to be alerted to these children well before the age of school entry. The community paediatrician who has the remit for children with special needs or neurodevelopmental problems will usually liaise with the appropriate education officer. Although it may vary between districts, this is usually the educational psychologist.

Summary

A basic definition of feeding is that it is, of course, fundamental to children's growth. If there is a feeding problem, of whatever cause, it is necessary to ensure that the child is getting adequate nutrition, that feeding is safe, efficient, comfortable and enjoyable. Feeding is also a core parenting and nurturing task, which, if it is not going well, can cause parents to feel undermined in their most basic of human roles, namely loving their child. One of the tasks of the community paediatrician is to ensure that the appropriate services are offered and put in place, not only to maximise the child's nutrition and growth but also to support the parents in this most fundamental and important of tasks.

References

Apgar V (1953) A proposal for a new method of evaluation of the newborn infant. *Current Research in Anaesthesiology.* **32**: 360.

Bax M (1998) Models and need. *Developmental Medicine and Child Neurology.* **40**: 291.

Berwick DM, Levy JC and Kleinerman R (1982) Failure to thrive: diagnostic yield of hospitalisation. *Archives of Diseases in Childhood.* **57**: 347–51.

Clayden GS (1992) Management of chronic constipation. *Archives of Diseases in Childhood.* **67**: 340–4.

Elthami M and Sullivan PB (1997) Nutritional management of the disabled child: the role of percutaneous endoscopic gastrostomy. *Developmental Medicine and Child Neurology.* **39**: 66–8.

Heine RG, Reddihough DS and Catto-Smith AG (1995) Gastroesophageal reflux and feeding problems after gastrostomy in children with severe neurological impairment. *Developmental Medicine and Child Neurology.* **37**: 320–9.

Larnert G and Ekberg O (1995) Positioning improves the oral and pharyngeal swallowing function in children with cerebral palsy. *Acta Paediatrica.* **84**: 689–92.

Newton RW and Wraith JE (1995) Investigation of developmental delay. *Archives of Diseases in Childhood.* **72**: 460–5.

Smith DW and Gong DT (1973) Scalp hair patterning as a clue to early fetal brain development. *Journal of Pediatrics.* **83**: 374–80.

Tawfik R, Dickson A, Clarke M and Thomas AG (1997) Caregivers' perceptions following gastrostomy in severely disabled children with feeding problems. *Developmental Medicine and Child Neurology.* **39**: 746–51.

Appendix: Support for parents

Financial

If appropriate, the community paediatrician will advise that the parents apply for the Disability Living Allowance (DLA). This may already have been suggested by other professionals involved with the child's care.

At the time of writing, the DLA is a tax-free social security benefit. It provides three rates of help, highest rate, middle rate and lowest rate, for personal care. Further information is available from the Benefits Enquiry Line (tel: 0800 882200).

A child aged three months or over may be able to get DLA because of their illness or disability because they:

- need help with washing, dressing, using the toilet, etc.
- need someone to keep an eye on them
- need someone with them when they are on kidney dialysis.

The community paediatrician would be expected to furnish reports detailing the child's condition when requested to do so by the Benefits Agency.

Invalid care allowance is a benefit which can be paid to people aged 16–65 years who are spending at least 35 hours a week caring for a severely disabled person who is in receipt of the middle or highest rate of DLA.

A variety of benefits is also available for those on low income. The community paediatrician may recommend that the involvement of a social worker would be helpful, particularly in the case of children with complex needs. The social worker could then advise which benefits the family may be entitled to. Alternatively, the family may approach the social security office or one of a number of voluntary advisory centres.

If the feeding problem is part of a more complex disability, the family may apply to the Family Fund Trust. The Family Fund Trust may make one-off payments for equipment, such as a washing machine, or for other needs, such as driving lessons to enable a parent to drive so a child can be taken to hospital appointments, etc. more easily. Further information can be obtained from the Family Fund Trust, PO Box 50, York YO1 2ZX (tel: 01904 621115).

A variety of charities may operate locally and assist with equipment such as wheelchairs, etc.

Respite

Many parents of children with complex disabilities want 'respite'. That is, a period of time when someone else is looking after their child and the parents have a break from childcare. This is less often required by parents of children whose sole difficulty is feeding.

The respite may take a variety of forms: it may be that another carer(s) looks after the child for a day a week; an overnight stay; a weekend stay; a week's stay. This may be away from the child's home at either a foster carer's home or at a local authority venue. Alternatively someone may come into the child's home and look after the child there, particularly if the child needs special equipment, such as lifting aids. The community paediatrician will ask local social services to arrange this if the parents wish (this may be through the generic social worker or through the disability team if there is one).

Nursery/playgroup

It is often helpful for young children with feeding difficulties to attend nursery. This has several advantages, including experience of playing and socialising with other children of the same age, and seeing them eat in an age-appropriate manner; if the parents can leave the child, this is a break for the parents (cf. respite); it provides an opportunity for the representatives of the education department (usually the educational psychologist) to observe the child.

Support groups

Support groups exist for a variety of syndromes, or occasionally specific conditions. These are often run by parents of children with that syndrome, with the aim of offering support and advice to parents, giving information to parents and professionals, and lobbying for more research and better resources. The quality of the information support groups provide is variable; the parents actively involved in many support groups may be without professional supervision; and there is usually no professional accountability.

Some parents find these groups very helpful, while others do not. Parents should be offered the details of the support group appropriate to their child's condition or situation, but then allowed to make the decision as to whether they make contact with the support group. The parents' names and contact details should never be passed to the support group without the parents' permission.

CHAPTER 3

Behavioural approaches to the assessment and management of feeding problems in young children

Jo Douglas

Introduction

Eating and feeding problems in young children are a common presenting problem in community settings and in acute care. Richman *et al.* (1982) found that 16% of three-year-olds were considered to have poor appetite and 12% were thought to be faddy by their parents, while a major survey of five-year-olds found that over one third were described retrospectively by their parents as having mild to moderate eating or appetite problems. Of this group, two thirds were described as 'faddy' (Butler and Golding 1986). Childhood eating problems account for approximately 25–35% of referrals to outpatient paediatric clinics in North America (Archer and Szatmari 1990) and up to 5% of paediatric hospital admissions (Wittenberg 1990).

There is a wide range of presentation of eating and feeding problems, from children who are severely underweight and failing to thrive to children who are faddy eaters. Some children have difficulty with textures of food, while others drink excessively. It is possible to adopt a psychological, psychiatric or medical framework. An attempt to group the different types of presentation has produced a descriptive, psychological model, which focuses on symptomatology rather than aetiology:

- problem with quantity, i.e. disinterest, poor appetite, food avoidance
- problem with texture, i.e. inappropriate texture for age
- problem with range, i.e. selective and faddy eaters (Douglas 1995b).

This type of classification can lead directly to ideas on management strategies in treatment.

Chatoor (1997) has followed an interactional model and suggested that feeding disorders should be assessed by evaluating the relationship between the infant and primary care-giver. She has outlined three developmental feeding disorders associated with failure to thrive:

- feeding disorder of homeostasis, i.e. poor reciprocity between infant and mother leading to inadequate food intake and irregular feeding pattern
- feeding disorder of attachment, i.e. poor attachment behaviours by mother and infant leading to inadequate food intake
- feeding disorder of separation, i.e. conflicts around autonomy between infant and mother leading to inadequate intake and extreme food selectivity.

In addition she suggests post-traumatic feeding disorder, which can occur at any stage of feeding development and occurs particularly when children have had aversive experiences with eating (Chatoor *et al.* 1988).

It is also possible to describe feeding problems on the basis of their quantifiable characteristics, i.e. total or partial food refusal, food selectivity by type or texture, swallowing disorder or conditioned dysphagia, meal-time tantrums or disruptive behaviour, tube-feeding dependence, rumination and vomiting, absence of self-feeding skills, excessive meal duration, adipsia and polydipsia (Babbit *et al.* 1994).

O'Brien *et al.* (1991) have suggested a taxonomy that includes cause, skill area and inappropriate behaviour. The causes may be environmentally independent (i.e. physically related) or dependent (i.e. behaviourally related). The skill areas include eating, self-feeding and social behaviour, while inappropriate behaviours are specific to each skill area. They suggest that treatment selection needs to be linked to the variables that control the behaviour and that such a taxonomy can help develop an approach for the systematic selection of treatment strategies.

Assessment of children's eating and feeding problems

Historically in the literature, there has been a dichotomy between organic and non-organic failure to thrive. But it has become progressively more clear to clinicians working in paediatrics that this is often a false dichotomy and that a mixed category that combines both of these factors is more helpful (Douglas 1995a; Skuse 1985; Wittenberg 1990). A recent study indicated that 26% of paediatric feeding disorder cases were attributable to organic factors, 10% to functional factors and 64% to both (Budd *et al.* 1992).

The biological context

Given the importance of organic factors in the aetiology of feeding difficulties, it is important for many of the children to have a paediatric assessment prior to referral for psychological intervention. A detailed medical history is essential in order to identify any significant factors in the development of the problem (*see* Chapter 2). This is particularly important if the child is vomiting, having bowel difficulties or repeated ENT/chest infections at the time of referral. Prematurity and intrauterine growth retardation are also significant risk factors. It possible that feeding difficulties may be yet another comorbid feature of prematurity (as discussed in Chapter 1).

Those offering psychological interventions should be fully aware of the background medical history as this will often provide the context for the aetiology of the feeding problem. Organic factors can have a considerable impact on the development of children's early eating patterns. Experiences of nausea, pain, choking, gagging or vomiting, if paired repeatedly with food and feeding, will eventually create the conditions for a conditioned association through the process of classical conditioning. Children with a wide range of medical conditions can experience this process. Douglas and Bryon (1996) found that in a feeding programme based in a paediatric hospital, 76% of the young children referred had been diagnosed with at least one significant medical problem in their early history. The range of medical problems included referrals from most paediatric specialities. Gastrointestinal problems, including gastro-oesophageal reflux and slow stomach emptying, feature extremely frequently, but in addition surgical patients who have pyloric stenosis, hiatus hernia, tracheo-oesophageal fistula or short gut syndrome are all at risk (Linscheid *et al.* 1987). Children with ENT problems may have experienced gagging or choking due to anatomical abnormalities, excessively large tonsils or poor oral-motor coordination. Immunological problems that lead to food allergies and sensitivities or poor resistance to illness can result in feeding problems.

Children with neurological impairments may have difficulties with oral-motor coordination or have developmental delays, which again are highly correlated with feeding difficulties. Other specialities that treat children with frequent presentation of eating problems include respiratory medicine (cystic fibrosis), nephrology (chronic renal failure) and cardiology. The specific problems faced by children with chronic conditions are discussed in Chapter 13.

Disruption to the normal developmental process of learning to eat may have long-lasting effects. Illingworth and Lister (1964) have proposed a 'critical period' between six and seven months of age when children easily acquire the ability to eat textured, solid foods. When there are circumstances that prevent this occurring naturally, they propose that it is considerably more difficult to establish oral feeding at a later age.

In addition to the medical history, a detailed feeding history will reveal the age at onset and the developmental pattern of the feeding process. Douglas and Bryon (1996) found that over half the mothers referred to their feeding clinic described their infants' distress while feeding during the first three months of life. Weaning on to baby purée and later on to lumpy, mashed food were also reported as times of considerable difficulty (Ramsay and Zelazo 1988).

If a child has been tube-fed then the duration and pattern of tube-feeding are also critical. The quantity of oral intake during the period of tube-feeding will influence the child's later ability to cope with tastes and textures. The diurnal pattern of tube-feeding can also influence the possibility of introducing eating. Daytime bolus feeding will impact significantly on the child's appetite and it will be far more difficult to interest the child in tasting and licking new flavours and foods when they feel satiated by the bolus feed. Overnight tube-feeding via a pump provides greater opportunity during the day for the child to feel hunger and associate the taste of foods with pleasurable sensations.

The child's height and weight measurements are required not only for percentile comparisons at assessment but also to relate to the child's past measurements. Tracking the point at which the child's weight started to fall down the centiles is important in understanding the history of the problem. Weight may have been low from birth or may have demonstrated a fall at the introduction of solid foods. Children whose weight and height fall below the third percentile are considered to be failing to thrive and are of considerable concern. When weights are above this level, parents may be surprised that their child's eating problem is not impacting negatively on weight and their high levels of concern may be alleviated. Parents of selectively eating children may then be relieved to find out that their child is within normal limits for height and weight on the limited range of food they are eating. If weight is not of concern, then psychological intervention can be directed entirely at the behavioural eating problem. However, if the child is failing to thrive then psychological intervention must focus on increasing the child's weight as a primary consideration before changing the texture or range of foods that the child eats.

Social and emotional context

Psychosocial issues can be contributory to the problem either at an aetiological level or as maintaining factors. If the child has a significant medical history it is, at times, difficult to assess the relative contribution of psychosocial issues, but it is feasible to postulate that a parent who has endured the uncertainty and anxiety of illness in an infant can often feel undermined in their parenting role. Difficulties with attachment to an ill infant or loss of opportunity to build up self-confidence in parenting in the early months may be critical and affect later parent–child attachment for many years (*see* Chapter 4). The experience of caring for a child who refuses to eat or is a poor eater because of undiagnosed or untreated gastro-oesophageal reflux or poor oral-motor coordination can undermine the parents' ability, confidence and self-esteem and consequently affect their parenting skills. Mothers frequently describe their sense of helplessness and also their confusion and lack of understanding about their child's feeding difficulties. 'Learned helplessness' in the parent may be an aetiological factor triggered by an infant who is unresponsive to or avoidant of feeding times.

Providing nutrition to a child is one of the most basic forms of care that a parent can provide and when the child refuses to cooperate this can attack the parents' emotional state at the core. The child's continued rejection of food can be experienced as rejection by the parent and so feelings of desperation, frustration and depression can build up. Advice received from health professionals may contribute to these feelings as the child's weight falls down the centiles. Exhortations from clinicians to feed the child and increase his or her weight are additional pressures and create unacceptable levels of anxiety in parents when no advice or help is provided to indicate how to encourage the child to eat more. Often the only way the parent can see is to force the child to feed, and sometimes this is inappropriately condoned by health professionals. Forcing the child to feed against their will by restricting the child's arms, forcing the bottle, teat or spoon into his or her mouth, slapping the child's face to precipitate crying and mouth-opening, or holding the child's nose can only compound the situation leading to more distress and anxiety for both parent and child. At times this behaviour may be reinforced by the child actually taking small quantities but it is not an approach that can be maintained over the long term by parents. It can also disguise the severity of the problem from health professionals who may consider that the child is growing and gaining weight at a rate sufficient to avoid further investigations or treatment.

Equally important is the state of the parental emotional and mental health regardless of the child's physical state. A mother who is chronically depressed cannot provide the care and attention a young infant requires to develop and grow. Her non-contingent responses will result in a poor ability to recognise the child's cues for hunger or stimulation. The child in turn can then become apathetic and withdrawn as attempts at stimulating the mother's response result either in an aversive interaction or no interaction at all. The child then gives up. Mothers who have a post-partum depression, who had poor parenting themselves as children or who are in dysfunctional relationships with their partner are at considerable risk (Pound *et al.* 1985). Assessing the mother's emotional state is therefore an essential part of the assessment process. Her support networks will indicate whether she has anyone to turn to for support and advice both practically and emotionally. Social isolation is an important contributory factor in mothers feeling abandoned, overstressed or depressed (Brown and Harris 1978).

Ethnic and cultural factors are also important, as some mothers from ethnic minorities may feel isolated due to language difficulties, cultural expectations that do not allow them out without their husbands, and no social contact with other mothers of the same cultural group. At times, a close family network may exist but this may compound rather than alleviate the situation if there is an overbearing grandmother or the mother is treated with contempt by in-laws.

High levels of anxiety can be as disruptive to parenting as depression. Mothers may find themselves drawn into conflict with their child about food and self-feeding. A mother's anxiety about her child's food intake may result in not allowing the child to self-feed at the appropriate age because of concern that the child will not eat enough. Concern and anxiety about cleanliness or obsessional concerns about mess can severely disrupt the child's normal developmental experience with touching food and learning to self-feed. A mother who will not let her child touch food in order to self-feed at the appropriate age because of concern about mess may communicate her anxiety to the child, who in turn becomes anxious about having sticky fingers. Mothers who continually wipe their child's hands or face while eating can also produce the same effect. Battles over the spoon can culminate in the child refusing to spoon feed from the mother.

Anxiety about the quantity the child is eating can distort the parent–child relationship. Parents will try to get the child to eat throughout the day and have no time for play and enjoyment. Mothers often describe how the constant pressure of thinking what to offer the child, buying it, preparing it and trying to get the child to eat it can take up all of their time. Offering a wide variety of meals and being prepared to cook three or four different meals in an effort to entice the child to eat can contribute to the child having an inappropriate level of control and becoming progressively more selective.

A mother's emotional state may also be affected by her own interpersonal relationships. Marital tension and dissatisfaction can create significant effects on maternal mental health by affecting her own sense of confidence and self-esteem.

Mothers' own attitudes to food and eating can also be relevant. Stein *et al.* (1994) have demonstrated that mothers with eating disorders show distorted patterns of feeding their own children. Mothers who have unusual attitudes to food, e.g. are overly concerned about fatty food or who are on special diets themselves, may also replicate these concerns in their child's diet.

Learning history

From a behavioural perspective it is important to consider the impact of the child's medical history and the family social and emotional history on the child's learning. Four routes of learning can contribute to the development of serious feeding difficulties in these children.

- Classical or stimulus conditioning in the child. Aversive conditioning will occur when the child experiences repeated pairing of physically unpleasant sensations with feeding. The learned association then creates food avoidance and refusal. The sight of food, the high chair or feeding utensils can eventually elicit behaviours of nausea, retching, vomiting and gagging without there being any organic reason for the behaviours.
- Operant conditioning in the child. Avoidant conditioning will occur when refusal to eat or drink is reinforced. The child may succeed in food being removed from them and efforts to get them to eat are terminated or they may gain parental attention for food refusal. Some children will be offered a range of preferred foods when they refuse food, tantrum or show aggressive behaviour.
- A combination of classical and operant conditioning in the child. This can occur when the child who has a classically conditioned avoidance of food is reinforced for pushing the food away by anxiety reduction or escape from eating (Linscheid *et al.* 1995).
- Skill deficit in the child. Lack of opportunity or physical deficits, e.g. oral-motor incoordination, can create a distortion in the developmental learning process of how to eat. Long-term tube-feeding may interfere with the normal developmental progression of eating, or parental behaviour can disrupt the child's opportunities to experience a full range of foods and textures. Parents who are anxious about their child choking may keep their child on puréed foods for an inappropriate length of time. Oral-motor delay can also affect the child's development of age-appropriate skills for eating and can be seen as creating a skill deficit-based problem (Babbitt *et al.* 1994).

These routes also affect the parents' learning and behaviour.

- Classical or stimulus conditioning in the parent. Repeated pairing of anxiety and stress while feeding a difficult child can create parental feelings of helplessness, anger, anxiety, rejection or withdrawal over time. The parental emotions elicited by trying to feed the child may still occur even when the child is no longer experiencing significant medical complications. The parent may continue with inappropriate patterns of behaviour based on their previous conditioned learning experiences.
- Operant conditioning in the parent. When the parent removes food from a child who is refusing food and crying, their behaviour is reinforced by the cessation of the child's distress. At times 'superstitious' behaviour will develop when the parents experience that the child eats with a particular spoon or bowl and then always assumes that the child will be unable to eat unless those specific eating utensils are involved. Parents of selectively eating children are highly reinforced for offering the same limited range of foods because the child eats them and gradually they stop offering other foods in an attempt to widen the child's range. When attempting to change

this behaviour pattern in parents the therapist needs to be aware of how strong the operant learning process is and how difficult it is to change when the parents are doubly reinforced by not having a crying, oppositional child at the table and by having a child who also eats food that is placed in front of them.

- Cognitive-behavioural learning in the parent. In addition to the stimulus–behaviour–consequence pattern of classical and operant conditioning, it is important to take into account parental cognitions about their child's behaviour. Their thoughts become mediators between the objective events, their subjective reaction and their responses. Parents will perceive their child's lack of eating in particular ways and make attributions about their behaviour in an attempt to understand it. Their attributions may be internal, e.g. 'He's not eating because he doesn't like me/I'm a hopeless mother', or external, e.g. 'He's not eating because he has something wrong with him medically/ he's naughty'. In a minority of extreme cases inaccurate attributions may become overgeneralised or may magnify certain of the child's behaviours to a distorted level. This can lead some parents to pursue inappropriate medical investigations of their child, while others feel depressed and detached from their infant whom they perceive as rejecting. Parents generally have the attribution that feeding their child is part of being a good parent. The discordance and stress that are evoked when the child refuses food and therefore does not allow the parent to be a 'good parent' can be extreme. Some parents can cope with this experience better than others, but the therapist must be aware of the development of negative self-attributions. A continual process of anxiously offering and removing food is often established with the parents not being effective in encouraging the child to feed. Some parents try offering wide ranges of food, frequently cooking several meals in an attempt to get their child to eat and may be intermittently reinforced by the child occasionally eating something.

- A combination of classical and operant conditioning in the parent. This occurs when a parent has experienced the continued stress of feeding an infant who refuses food in the early months of life and who is reinforced by reduction of anxiety about the child's weight when the child feeds under force. In other cases, the anxiety about weight loss caused by early food refusal in selective eaters is reinforced by reduction of anxiety when the child drinks a lot of milk or eats a lot of strictly selected groups of foods. Unusual behaviours occur with parents allowing their children to drink six pints of milk a day or eat four packets of biscuits and ten yoghurts. Parents whose anxiety has been reduced by tube-feeding their child may be very reluctant to give up the tube when the child can eventually eat orally.

- Lack of knowledge about eating and diet – a skill deficit in the parents. Many parents need advice and help to offer their child an appropriate range of foods. A child who is underweight needs to have food that is high in calories, i.e. contains a lot of fats or sugars. A parent who persists in feeding low-fat yoghurt to a child who is failing to thrive needs specific instructions and monitoring about what he or she is offering the child to eat. Parents may need help in understanding their child's oral-motor problems and how to offer the appropriate textures for the child to eat. Teaching a child to chew and swallow may be a whole new area of learning.

Existing patterns of eating

Although the child's medical and emotional history is important in understanding the aetiological influences, it is vital to assess the existing pattern of eating by direct observation of the parents and child at a meal time. This observation provides a wealth of information about existing maintaining factors. Meal-time observation can be in the home, for a more naturalistic setting, or in the clinic.

The physical setting for meals can be immensely varied, with some children sitting on their parent's lap, some tightly strapped into a high chair, while others are often observed to run freely around the room with the parent following in pursuit with a spoonful of food. The use of appropriate foods and eating utensils can influence the child's eating, as can the child's demands for particular spoons or bowls. The setting conditions for eating need to be clear and consistent for the child, with the child feeling physically contained and safe with easy access to the food within reach. A pattern of meal-time presentation on a regular basis rather than grazing and snacking throughout the day can use hunger and satiation cycles to best advantage and help the child recognise the reinforcing feelings associated with eating.

The child's behaviour during the meal may demonstrate a strong avoidance reaction with crying, signs of fear and a desire to escape being shown as soon as food is brought within sight. The food refusal may be maintained by negative reinforcement when the refusal to eat terminates the parents' demands. Other children may react with interest and positive comments when presented with food but then only eat a couple of spoonfuls before they stop and want to get down. The child's desire and ability to try different types and textures of food, to self-feed, to touch food and let themselves get messy, to concentrate and persevere with eating, and to demand the parents' attention during the meal are all clearly identifiable during an observation and need to be related to the parents' behaviour.

The parents' behaviour during the meal will demonstrate the strategies they regularly use to encourage their child to eat. Some will distract their child by reading a book or giving them toys to play with while they feed them. Others will try to force their child to accept the spoon or the bottle. The timing of the parents' attention, encouragement and praise in relation to eating will provide the basis of a functional analysis. Parents are often ineffectual with their attempts to get their child to eat, they often continually question the child, they may be inconsistent in their requests and do not carry through what they say. Some parents may be very passive, uninvolved and distant during the meal, while others are over-involved and anxious, pressurising the child and interfering with their attempts to self-feed. These observations contribute to the functional analysis, which is the basis of behavioural intervention. It attempts to identify the contingent relationships between the parents' and the child's behaviour and identifies features of the parents' behaviour that serve as antecedents and consequences for the child's feeding behaviour.

More formal observational measures are also possible. Babbitt *et al.* (1994) describe objective measures in an observational schedule in their programme in Maryland. They individually tailor a standard baseline assessment for each child and use a detailed list of operationally defined behaviours for self-feeding and non-self-feeding children. The amount the child consumes is recorded as frequency counts of bites or drinks taken of each food or drink per minute. Inappropriate behaviour, such as dawdling, negative comments or distraction, is recorded using an interval sampling procedure, i.e. recording occurrence and non-occurrence of the behaviour. Pre- and post-meal weights of the food and drinks are taken and the numbers of grams consumed are calculated. Target behaviours can be specified in considerable detail, e.g. a bit of food can be operationally defined as the child opening his or her mouth within five seconds of food presentation.

Behavioural approaches to treating feeding problems

The basis of any operant behavioural management approach is to remove contingent reinforcers that are maintaining the inappropriate behaviour and provide them contingently for appropriate behaviour. Management of a classically conditioned behaviour focuses on the reduction of anxiety elicited by the stimuli of food in order to encourage approach and consumption of the food (Palmer *et al.* 1975).

These two behavioural approaches are often combined in children, particularly where both processes of learning have occurred. Children need the opportunity to unlearn their fear and parents need help and instructions about how to support their children through that process.

Reduction of anxiety in children

Desensitisation approaches can be used with food-phobic children to help them eventually eat the target food. Children who are worried about mess on their hands can gradually learn to tolerate touching wet or sloppy foods during self-feeding by teaching them through a process of play to touch different non-food textures and eventually graduating on to food. Children who are selective eaters may show terror at being encouraged to try a non-preferred food but may be able to take a tiny crumb of a new food and gradually overcome their fear by eating graduated amounts. When children have become avoidant of their high chairs because of the association with unpleasant eating experiences, they can overcome their fears by having short opportunities to play with toys while seated in the high chair. As their fear reduces, plates, bowls and cutlery, and eventually food, can be reintroduced. Children who have a fear of drinking can take the first steps to overcoming this by playing in the bath and sucking from a sponge or a flannel and gradually learning that drinking water can be fun. Pairing an anxiety-producing stimulus with the relaxed association of play can help young, pre-school children overcome their fear. Children who have never taken food orally can become familiar with food initially by playing with and handling it. Gradual encouragement and modelling how to take small licks from fingers and utensils will start to overcome the child's avoidance and unfamiliarity. A combination of operant and classical conditioning approaches, involving decreasing the anxiety and using positive reinforcement, can be most successful.

A structured and graded approach to texture of food will also enable children to eat more appropriate textures for their age. Children who have never eaten solids will need to progress through the stages of puréed, mashed, chopped, bite/dissolve, semi-solid and solid foods. Children who are fixed on a stage of puréed food at an inappropriate age will also need help to build up their confidence and ability to eat more textured foods.

Reduction of anxiety in parents

Many parents experience high levels of distress and anxiety when their child does not eat. This can lead to many inappropriate management methods being used. Reduction of parental distress is essential if they are to carry out a change programme. Parents who are overly concerned about their child's weight will need the reassurance of regular weight checks and to understand the centile charts. If the child is failing to thrive then tube-feeding via a nasogastric tube can be an important alternative to oral feeding and can significantly reduce parental anxiety while they build up their child's confidence with food and eating. Tube-feeding needs to be carried out overnight in this instance so that the child has the opportunity to feel some hunger in the day and benefit from the opportunities to play with food and taste it in small amounts with no pressure or expectation.

Parents can be helped to reduce their anxiety by providing them with appropriate dietary information about high-calorie foods so that they can maximise the calorific value of each mouthful that their child eats. In addition, ideas about what foods to offer their child and discussion of menus can help reduce the strain they feel and the loneliness of coping on their own.

Many parents will have tried to force feed. It is essential that this approach is always stopped as it will only exacerbate the problem. Distracting the child with toys or television while they spoon in the food is a method that parents often develop to cope with children who will not eat. But their anxiety is aroused when this fails to work as the child starts to resist being fed, loses interest in the toy or programme, or grows older, and the parents become concerned that their child is not self-feeding.

Encouraging self-feeding and participation in feeding can be an anxiety-provoking time for parents. They lose control over the amount they can spoon into the child, they see less food going in as the child is not as efficient or effective as they are, and they have to cope with the mess. Parents who are fastidious about cleanliness can find the process of teaching a child to self-feed unbearable. They tend to keep wiping the child's hands and face during the meal, which causes irritation and interrupts the child's pattern of eating. Parents can easily communicate their anxiety about mess to the child, who then learns not to touch food and becomes upset by the slightest bit of food on their hands. Supporting parents during this process is essential if the child is going to make the necessary developmental progress with self-feeding. Modelling with the parents how to encourage their child to self-feed and touch food can be a supportive approach.

Working with parents to overcome their child's feeding problem in a manner that is supportive and not critical is essential if they are to gain in confidence in their parenting. They need to understand the reasons for the change in their approach but not to feel blamed for the problem. They need to see small steps of success in order to continue and they need continual reassurance and support that they are progressing on the correct route for change to occur. Prescriptive advice rarely works unless the parents fully accept it and have the reserves of energy and dedication to carry it through. More frequently, provision of regular help to monitor their progress and help them consider the next stage of change is required. They need to participate in a process of change in order to see change in their child's eating.

Teaching children to eat

Operant learning approaches provide powerful techniques when teaching new skills: positive reinforcement, modelling, shaping and fading. Contingent social attention is the most basic behavioural procedure. Positive attention, praise, hugs and claps can all be used effectively to encourage children to eat. Being clear about the goal of success is important so that the desired behaviour is socially reinforced (Hoch *et al.* 1994).

Other positive consequences or reinforcers can be stickers on charts, tokens, food pictures to stick in a scrap book, access to television (Bernal 1972), opportunity to play with toys, access to a preferred food or sensory stimulation (Luiselli and Gleason 1987). The Premack Principle is also a positive reinforcement strategy that is of value in certain cases of selective eating, i.e. access to the preferred food is made contingent on acceptance of a non-preferred food (Bernal 1972).

Stimulus control techniques can be used to help overcome the avoidance of food. Shaping and fading are two commonly used techniques. Shaping helps the child approximate closer and closer approaches to the feared stimulus. Reinforcing a child to come to the table, then sit down at the table to eat can take a number of stages until the child can sit for the duration of a meal. Teaching a child to eat a larger portion or to eat a non-preferred food can progress in small stages by gradually increasing the quantity of the new food that the child is expected to eat every few days. Similarly, helping a child progress through textures of food requires a combination of gradual texture change plus social reinforcement and access to preferred textures. These children sometimes require additional teaching to know how to chew rather than attempting to swallow lumps. Demonstrating how to chew and swallow, and helping the child learn to clear his or her mouth at each mouthful before taking in the next mouthful are all necessary learned skills of eating.

Encouraging self-feeding requires physical prompts initially, with reciprocal behaviour between the parents and child. Battles over the spoon are to be avoided, but the child may not be fully capable of total self-feeding and so a process of the parents helping in loading and guiding the spoon may be essential until the child's physical skills mature.

Removing unwanted behaviours

Extinction and negative reinforcement are valuable approaches in some instances.

Parents may need training to recognise when they are providing attention for non-eating and disruptive behaviour rather than eating (Stark *et al.* 1990;

Turner *et al.* 1994). It is often easy to observe excessive parental efforts to encourage the child to eat which appear to have diminishing returns in effectiveness. Yet if the child does eat appropriately parents often ignore the child for fear of interrupting or disrupting the desired behaviour. Training parents to use their social attention discriminately can often be a successful strategy. But if a child is readily throwing food around the room then parents will need to stop the behaviour by indicating their displeasure to the child.

When an infant has vomited frequently or over long periods of time, some parents become highly sensitised to their child's signals. They will avoid confronting the child about food or other behavioural issues in case he or she vomits and loses all of the meal that they have just taken great efforts to get into the child. This can lead to the child always getting his or her own way and becoming too powerful in the relationship. Parents require encouragement to exert the appropriate level of behavioural boundaries for their child without being held to ransom by threats of vomit. If self-induced retching, gagging or vomiting is suspected then the parents need to learn how to set clear limits for their child and ignore the threatened behaviour. If the child does proceed, the parent can either demand that the child eats the same food or twice as much food again, so that the child does not gain reinforcement from the behaviour. This can be a stressful experience for the parents, but once they realise that it works it usually only has to be carried out a few times before the child learns that the behaviour is not effective.

In general, extinction, time out and negative reinforcement approaches are not useful strategies for young children with severe feeding difficulties. A threat to remove the food and throw it away is often precisely what the child desires and so it is very important for the parent to understand clearly what is a positive or a negative reinforcer for their child.

Changing parental cognitions and attributions

Many parents change their attributions very rapidly once the child starts to show small signs of progress, but some parents' cognitions will interfere with the possibility of change and they will be resistant to interventions that do not match their attributions, e.g. a parent who feels inappropriately that her child needs a particular medical investigation will not be cooperative in using behavioural management techniques, and a parent who feels that their child is naughty will have difficulty using positive reinforcment. The therapist needs to be aware of where the resistance to change is based and enable the parents to adopt alternative views, develop problem-solving strategies and correct cognitive errors.

Parents' expectations of change may also be unrealistic in terms of pace or goal. The therapist will need to set the framework and expectations for change and enable the parents to modify their views. Regular contact with the parents and positive feedback about the rate of change and the small steps of success are critical for this to be effective.

Conclusions

A cognitive behavioural framework is useful in the assessment, classification and treatment of children's feeding problems. As with any parent training approach to behaviour problems, parents need help and guidance in how to carry out these strategies with their children. The context of the feeding difficulty needs to be understood and factors that are maintaining the child's problems need to be identified. The stresses and strains on the parents must be fully recognised in order to intervene most effectively.

Severe and chronic childhood feeding problems frequently develop in relation to the physical experiences of the child. This creates a learning environment which may perpetuate long after the original stimulus is no longer present. Analysis of maintaining factors is essential for successful treatment to occur. Techniques that address the anxiety generated both in the child and the parents, as well as reinforcing positive steps to change, can be very successful.

References

Archer LA and Szatmari P (1990) Assessment and treatment of food aversion in a four year old boy: a multi-dimensional approach. *Canadian Journal of Psychiatry.* **35**: 501–5.

Babbit RL, Hoch TA, Coe DA *et al.* (1994) Behavioural assessment and treatment of paediatric feeding disorders. *Journal of Developmental and Behavioural Paediatrics.* **15**: 278–91.

Bernal ME (1972) Behavioural treatment of a child's eating problem. *Journal of Behaviour Therapy and Experimental Psychiatry.* **3**: 43–50.

Brown G and Harris T (1978) *Social Origins of Depression.* Tavistock, London.

Budd KS, McGraw TE, Farbisz R *et al.* (1992) Psychosocial concomitants of children's feeding disorders. *Journal of Paediatric Psychology.* **17**: 81–92.

Butler NR and Golding J (eds) (1986) *From Birth to Five: a study of health and behaviour in Britain's five year olds.* Pergamon, London.

Chatoor I (1997) Feeding disorders of infants and toddlers. In: JD Noshpitz (ed)

Handbook of Child and Adolescent Psychiatry, vol. 1, pp. 367–86. John Wiley, New York.

Chatoor I, Conley C and Dickson L (1988) Food refusal after an incident of choking: a post traumatic eating disorder. *Journal of the American Academy of Child and Adolescent Psychiatry*. **27**: 105–10.

Douglas J (1995a) Behavioural eating disorders in young children. *Current Paediatrics*. **5**: 39–42.

Douglas J (1995b) Types of behavioural eating problems in young children. In: DP Davies (ed) *Nutrition in Child Health*. Royal College of Physicians of London, BPA, London.

Douglas J and Bryon M (1996) Interview data on severe behavioural eating difficulties in young children. *Archives of Diseases in Childhood*. **75**: 304–8.

Hoch TA, Babbitt RL, Coe DA *et al.* (1994) Contingency contracting: combining positive reinforcement and escape extinction procedures to treat persistent food refusal. *Behavior Modification*. **18**: 106–28.

Illingworth RS and Lister J (1964) The critical or sensitive period, with special reference to certain feeding problems in infants and children. *Journal of Paediatrics*. **65**: 839–48.

Linscheid TR, Tarnowski KJ, Rasnake LK and Brams JS (1987) Behavioural treatment of food refusal in a child with short gut syndrome. *Journal of Pediatric Psychology*. **12**: 451–60.

Linscheid TR, Budd KS and Rasnake LK (1995) Pediatric feeding disorders. In: MC Roberts (ed) *Handbook of Pediatric Psychology*, (2e). Guilford Press, New York.

Luiselli JK and Gleason DJ (1987) Combining sensory reinforcement and texture fading procedures to overcome chronic food refusal. *Journal of Behavior Therapy and Experimental Psychology*. **18**: 149–55.

O'Brien S, Repp AC, Williams GE and Christopherson ER (1991) Pediatric feeding disorders. *Behavior Modification*. **15**: 394–418.

Palmer S, Thompson RJ and Linscheid TR (1975) Applied behavior analysis in the treatment of childhood feeding problems. *Developmental Medicine and Child Neurology*. **17**: 333–9.

Pound A, Cox A, Puckering C and Mills M (1985) The impact of maternal depression on young children. In: JE Stevenson (ed) *Recent Research in Developmental Psychopathology*. Pergamon, Oxford.

Ramsay M and Zelazo P (1988) Food refusal in failure to thrive infants: naso-gastric feeding combined with interactive-behavioral approach. *Journal of Pediatric Psychology*. **13**: 329–47.

Richman N, Stevenson J and Graham P (1982) *Pre-school to School: a behavioural study*. Academic Press, London.

Skuse D (1985) Non-organic failure to thrive: a reappraisal. *Archives of Diseases in Childhood*. **60**: 173–8.

Stark LJ, Bowen AM, Tyc VL *et al.* (1990) A behavioural approach to increasing calorie consumption in children with cystic fibrosis. *Journal of Pediatric Psychology.* **15**: 309–26.

Stein A, Woolley H, Cooper SD and Fairburn CG (1994) An observational study of mothers with eating disorders and their infants. *Journal of Child Psychology and Psychiatry.* **35**: 733–48.

Turner KMT, Sanders MR and Wall CR (1994) Behavioural parent training versus dietary education in the treatment of children with persistent feeding difficulties. *Behaviour Change.* **11**: 242–58.

Wittenberg JVP (1990) Feeding disorders in infancy: classification and treatment considerations. *Canadian Journal of Psychiatry.* **35**: 529–33.

CHAPTER 4

Feeding difficulties in infancy and childhood: psychoanalytic perspectives

Stephen Briggs

Introduction

This chapter applies a psychoanalytic perspective to the dynamics of feeding difficulties in childhood. Concentrating primarily on the early feeding relationship in infancy, theoretical formulations, particularly those originating in the object relations school, of the parent–infant relationship will be discussed. It is from this theoretical base that the distinctive dynamics of feeding difficulties within the parent–infant relationships are explored. It is demonstrated that the conscious and unconscious factors that affect parenting, and the development of characteristic patterns of relating between parents and infants, and in the infant's emerging character can be understood – and that this understanding has a distinctive quality – from a psychoanalytic perspective. The role of detailed observation in developing an understanding of the individual patterns of infant development is illustrated with examples, in the form of vignettes, from clinical practice and observation. The chapter then discusses the implications of feeding difficulties for the infant's future development, especially in the arenas of thinking, relating and symbolising, and it concludes by making some observations on how the psychoanalytic approach can inform professional intervention.

Parent–infant relationships in early infancy

The distinctive quality of psychodynamic approaches to feeding difficulties in infancy and childhood lies in the emphasis that is placed on understanding the emotional qualities of the feeding relationship. From the beginning of life the infant and the mother are engaged in a relationship which is emotionally significant for both, and which is complex. Winnicott suggested that:

> If you set out to describe a baby, you will find that you are describing a baby and someone else. A baby cannot exist alone, but is essentially part of a relationship (Winnicott 1964).

This can be said to be the point at which psychoanalytic theory of infant development began to concentrate, within the object relations tradition, on a two-person rather than a one-person psychology.

Recent attention to patterns of relationship in infancy and problems within the feeding relationship in infancy and childhood extend and develop ideas about both the infantile and the parental contributions to the quality of these relationships. On the one hand, the infant is seen as an active participant in the relationship, bringing to it the capacity to develop patterns of timing and rhythm in relationships (Alvarez 1992), and distinct and individual ways of communicating. On the other hand, conceptualisations of the mother's role in attending to and transforming the emotional experiences of the infant, particularly Bion's theory of the container–contained relationship (Bion 1962), have enabled developments in the study of parent–infant interactions from a psychoanalytic perspective.

Establishing a feeding relationship is a momentous experience for both mother and infant. Of course the infant brings to the relationship capacities which enhance the process, notably the sucking reflex and the capacity to indicate, through a range of communications, both the desire to be fed and the wish for proximity. The mother too brings both the desire to feed her infant, to establish a relationship with him or her, and also anxieties which reflect both the newness of the experience – even if this is not the first baby – and the responsibilities of the role.

As Daws (1995) describes it:

> Parents who have just had a baby are normally in a heightened state of emotion. Life and death feelings are part of the ordinary stuff of [infancy].

This 'heightened' state of emotion was thought by Winnicott (1965) to be a means whereby the mother, through 'primary maternal preoccupation', made a space in her mind for the arrival of her new baby and prepared herself for a kind of communication which of necessity depends upon pre- or non-verbal modes. Bion (1962) developed a similar idea in that he described the mother's state of readiness to receive infant communications as forming a kind of 'reverie'. Reverie comprises a state of mind in the mother in which she allows the baby's experiences to enter her mind, so that she can think about and gather a sense of the meaning of infantile communications. These are then used to formulate, consciously and unconsciously, responses to the infant's communications and needs. The parental capacity for reverie and primary maternal preoccupation depends upon the experience and internalisation of a similarly receptive mother in the mother's own infancy and childhood.

Emotions are heightened and extreme, and in these circumstances tend to 'spill out', requiring space and containment. The experience of the infant of early life is thought to have a particular kind of intensity, almost in a way which defies words, but which psychoanalytic theory has tried to put into words. The intense experiences of early infancy are described by the generic term 'primitive anxieties'. Winnicott writes of 'primitive agonies' (Winnicott 1974), and Bion of 'nameless dread', appropriately conjuring the idea that these feelings and experiences do not have names. Bick, like Winnicott, thought of the experiences of falling, of falling apart, as if 'liquefying' or 'falling for ever' (Bick 1986). The vulnerability of the infant in these moments is such that he or she is unable to hold within himself or herself the emotional experiences to which he or she is subject. He or she looks therefore, using primitive methods of communication, particularly projective identification (Klein 1946; Bion 1967), to a parent who can undertake, on his or her behalf, the emotional work of first allowing the infant's experiences to permeate her, making sense within herself of the infant's communications before responding to her baby, through her words, gestures and deeds. The infant then experiences the parental function as holding, integrating and helping the infant to form and remain within his or her own 'psychic skin'. The 'good enough' (Winnicott 1974) and 'balanced' (Bion 1967) mother, who is able to make sense of her own experiences of heightened emotion and communicate in this way with her infant, provides names for emotional experiences, which, through repetition, enable the infant to build within an internal world in which he or she has felt understood and can understand his or her own emotional experiences. Bion calls this the 'container–contained' relationship, a concept which has had a tremendous influence on psychoanalytic thinking and practice.

In psychoanalytic theory, the attempts to describe the heightened and extreme emotional field of infant–parent relationships reflect the intensity of these experiences as they are thought to be experienced by the mother and infant. Similarly, the experience of moments of integration, when being held or feeding, also requires a language which reflects the intensity of these experiences. What is at stake is not simply the amelioration of anxious moments, but the origins of intimacy and the capacity to develop intimate relationships. Through having a sense of timing and developing rhythms of interaction with her baby, through her reverie and understanding, the mother has the responsibility of making available to the infant a subjective world of shared meaning (Stern 1985).

It is useful therefore to think of early development as a configuration, not only of interactions between infant and mother, but also within each of them. The parental approach to the infant's needs and communications is influenced by current relationships, past experiences and, where feeding is concerned, the experiences – probably not remembered consciously – of the parent's own feeding as an infant. The patterns and attitudes that develop from all of these factors can be thought of as evidencing the internalised qualities of relationships in the parent. The infant not only brings a particular disposition to the world of relationships, but also, through intrauterine experiences, has a past (see, for example, Piontelli 1992). The advantages of thinking of development in terms of such a gestalt, or configuration, are that a complex epistemology with regard to change and growth is provided, and oversimplified solutions or stereotyping are eschewed; that each parent–infant/child relationship needs careful individual study, through observation, and that the professional has a range of possibilities to think about before reaching a conclusion in a particular case. This range of possibilities includes thinking about the parent, the infant/child and the quality of contact between them. Feeding, in this framework, is not just about the passing of physical nurture from one person to another, but rather about the communication of elemental aspects of intimacy – of love, hate and truth.

Increasingly, particularly in the field of child psychotherapy, psychoanalytic thinking is influenced by direct observation. A method of observation, where an infant and a young child are observed weekly in the home for one hour for a period of one or two years, is now an essential training experience (Bick 1964; Miller *et al.* 1989). This kind of observation has been extended in its application so that professionals from all disciplines undertake observation on all training courses in the Tavistock Clinic. Called the 'Tavistock Model' (Reid 1997), the method has been taken up by a wide range of training institutions (e.g. Briggs 1992; Tanner and Le Riche 1998). Recently, this form of observation has been developed as a research methodology (Rustin 1989, 1997; Briggs 1997). Closely detailed accounts of interaction and the behaviour and communications of the infant are encouraged in this essentially naturalistic method of observation. Open, unstructured descriptive accounts of mother–infant relationships are produced for discussion in seminar groups, and the observer develops qualities of reflectiveness based on openness to the emotionality in the setting. This reflective capacity is a precondition for the therapist developing 'reverie', to use Bion's term, mirroring the function of the mother and thus a willingness to remain in a state of 'not knowing' long enough to develop a sense of the impact of the emotionality in the relationship between mother and infant. The observer thus becomes equipped to make use of the feelings he or she has in the course of therapeutic work, the countertransference. Experienced practitioners use such observation training alongside their own experiences of analysis and therapy to develop the capacity to use feelings and reactions within themselves economically and creatively.

Feeding difficulties in infancy: an emphasis on parenting

Dilys Daws, in two papers (1993, 1997) which elegantly review her experiences of psychotherapy with parents and infants, explores the problems presented to her by parents who are concerned about their babies' feeding difficulties. Daws demonstrates the capacity the skilled therapist has to move, in his or her mind, through thinking about interactions between parent and infant, the internal experiences of both, and what happens inside himself or herself, the therapist. The therapist applies the open, reflective, observational approach to notice and make use of his or her own reactions.

Daws discusses the connections between the dynamics in the families and the impact of these families on her, the therapist. Working with parents and infants with feeding difficulties impacts on the worker with a range of emotions, 'from voracious greed to an inability to take in what is offered' (Daws 1993, p 75), and these feelings make sense of a particular part of the experiences within the family. She distinguishes between two kinds of feeding difficulty. On the one hand there are situations where the infant is underfed, leading to failure to thrive; on the other hand is a pattern where the infant is fed little and often, but both mother and infant become exhausted by the constant feeding cycle. While she does pay attention during the consultations with the families to the individual qualities of the infant, the emphasis in her work is on the different ways in which the parent is influenced by the impact of her baby, what is stirred up in the mother from the past, and the way this becomes patterned into her relationships with the infant and others. The two categories of feeding difficulty are best considered separately.

The infant who 'feeds too much' is a snack feeder. Here the mother may be responding to infant communications more at a physical level than an emotional one, and 'there is no shape to the meal as an emotional encounter' (p 73). From a number of examples from her consultations, Daws shows that the repeated snack feeding masks a deep-seated fear in the parent of separation, which often takes the form that the infant will die if separate (a response therefore to the problem of heightened emotion about life and death). Also, in these circumstances, the mother's own infantile feeding experiences have been stirred up by the experience of feeding her baby. Here, as Daws puts it, 'Mothers who endlessly feed their babies may also be expressing unending hunger in themselves and are not able to feel reciprocally fed and satisfied by their babies' satisfaction' (p 73).

Bereavements and other losses lay behind the problem in separating. In one case, which Daws cites, the mother had murderous feelings towards her own mother, which she denied to herself, and also a strong hostility towards any form of structure, including the structure of the therapy. The hatred of structure was found also in the feeding of her baby. In the kind of relationship between mother and infant which Daws is describing here, intimacy is not possible because, although there is a capacity for closeness, there is difficulty in being apart. Closeness is obtained at the cost of interpreting the infant's communications always as a wish for a feed. These two points – the significance of the parent responding to the infant not just at a physical level, but also through attending to the emotional meaning and relatedness of the baby, and the relationship between mother's early (and subsequent) relationships – can be developed further.

The idea that infants make and respond to communications at an emotional level is part of Klein's contribution to object relations theory. She wrote:

> 'I have seen babies as young as three weeks interrupt their sucking for a short time to play with mother's breast or look towards her face. I have also observed that young infants – even as early as the second month – would, in wakeful periods after feeding, lie on mother's lap, look up at her, listen to her voice and respond to it by their facial expression' (Klein 1952).

This observation of Klein's, made over 45 years ago, now seems to be really understating the case that infants have a capacity to relate in quite complex ways from birth. Current psychoanalytic thinking accords with developmental psychology with regard to the complexity of infantile relating, while differing with regard to emphasis. Difficulties in mothers who are unable to relate to young infants in a way that acknowledges their capacity for emotional interaction are attributable to many factors. On one level, it is a common fallacy that babies 'just eat and sleep'. This itself may be a defence against feelings which may be stirred up in the parent, who as an infant may in fact have been treated as someone who 'just ate and slept'. Socially, particular patterns of childcare, in particular settings of time and place, may reflect a structuring of defences against the impact of 'heightened' emotions, such as four-hourly feeding, leaving infants unattended at night (in cots) or in the day (in prams), leaving infants to cry (together with a rationalisation for this practice). Infant death must also be related to the heightened feelings of a life and death nature experienced emotionally by parents and infants in these early relationships.

Missed infantile communications or communications which are treated at a physical rather than an emotional level may also be the consequences of depression in the mother (Murray 1992) or of a mother's other troubling or difficult preoccupations. A combination of these factors, and a lack of confidence within the mother of being able to be guided by the qualities of the actual relationship she has with her baby can also lead to the mother turning away from the intimacy of direct communication with the baby. Martha Harris

(1975) gave an example from an observation of a mother who, in contrast, though feeling herself to be limited in some respects and aware of her own childhood difficulties, allowed herself to learn from experience with her baby, to be taught by her baby, so to speak. I myself have studied situations where mothers in difficult and stressful circumstances missed, or could not let themselves see and know about, the infant's emotional communications with them. One mother, Anne, a very underconfident mother, demonstrated the effect of this on her feeding the first time I saw her with her baby, Samantha. Samantha, at 13 days, was asleep in her mother's arms, then:

> Anne moved a little and Samantha, still asleep, moved with her so that her head was lying back, almost out of Anne's arms in a slightly unsupported way. Anne told me she felt a lot of pain after the Caesarean and this was the first day she had not thought about having a painkiller. Samantha stirred, opening her eyes slowly, quietly. She looked towards Anne's face. Anne said she was awake at last and said 'I'm just going to feed her'. She offered the right breast to Samantha and made a grimace as she took the nipple. She read-justed and Samantha lost the nipple, then took it again and sucked steadily. Anne sat cross-legged on the sofa, holding Samantha quite low down so that her face seemed to be hidden in Anne's top.

In this piece of interaction, Samantha is seeking mother with her eyes, demonstrating her wish to relate to her; mother took this to mean she wanted feeding. Samantha sucked steadily, making a good grip on the nipple. She was not perturbed by needing to start the feed twice. On the other hand, for mother Anne, the feed was preceded by her reporting pain from the childbirth and the process of making contact with Samantha was also painful; that is to say, she grimaced. As the feed progressed, Anne's conversation followed a wide range of subjects all of which seemed to reflect on her lack of confidence. She then returned to the subject of breast-feeding:

> Anne said she had found she was running out of milk by the evening, and Donald had always been hungry. She said that when Donald had been a baby she had not closed the curtains of the room which led to his waking at 4 am. Samantha stopped sucking, holding the nipple in her mouth and Anne looked down at her and then lifted her away from the breast and held her over her shoulder. Anne looked at her again and said 'you're hungry, that's what you are'. She said she thought she would go and make a bottle for Samantha.

Her lack of confidence in herself, in the face of her many preoccupations, is graphically illustrated in her turning to a bottle – as though she feels unable to feed Samantha from within herself. Feeding difficulties emerged in the form of a self-fulfilling prophecy, that Samantha was not satisfied by breast-feeding, and she regurgitated bottle feeds. Anne herself had a background in which she had experienced her mother as not able to feed her adequately.

The presence in any combination of lack of confidence, depression, anxiety about meeting the baby's needs, and preoccupation with troubling issues – in Anne's case her older child – can lead a mother to miss her baby's cues and to withdraw from relating to the baby. In an unusual observational example provided by Susan Reid (Reid 1997), a glimpse is obtained of the way a mother's own infantile feeding experiences can influence her feeding of her own baby. In these observations there is seen repeatedly a difficulty stemming from mother's apparent need to control the feeding situation:

> The observer noted feed after feed the way that mother firmly held on to the bowl and the spoon. The infant was never allowed to hold the spoon or touch her food, certainly not to play with it and explore its qualities.

This made the observation of feeds tense and difficult. The mother returned to work when the infant was six months old and the observations continued in the maternal grandmother's home. To the observer's amazement she found that the grandmother fed in an identical way to the infant's mother.

Reid comments:

> Of course the infant's mother had no conscious memory of this, but perhaps an unconscious blueprint had been made of the experience. It seemed to have survived totally unmodified (Reid 1997, p 10).

'Ghosts in the nursery' and failure to thrive

The impact on parents of early but consciously not remembered experiences, which, as Reid notes, have somehow remained unmodified by time and experience, can in some circumstances form 'ghosts in the nursery', to use Selma Fraiberg's term (Fraiberg 1980). Often, these experiences are of the impact of an actual, retrievable event, either from the recent or more distant past, which impacts on the parent and interferes with parenting. One of the mothers in my study appeared affected by a distant 'ghost' who was both known and unknown to her:

> Yvonne, the mother, made repeated references to the cot death of her younger brother when she was a small child. These references seemed unconnected in the way she told me about them from the current situation, in which she found herself in an aggressive and sometimes quite cruel relationship with her infant daughter, Hester,

her second child. Her fear of damaging her baby, of strangling her, or of hurting her in other ways suggested Yvonne's identification with a mother who could not keep babies alive and a murderous older sibling. Breast-feeding was ended prematurely so that neither she nor her son should know these feelings of jealousy of the new baby, Hester, who was repeatedly sick after feeds.

In this case the 'ghost in the nursery' is dimly remembered but creates a painful and difficult scenario for all the family. At times, the presence of a 'ghost' can be 'detected' with dramatic outcome. Brazelton and Cramer (1991) give a number of illustrations of how these events lead to the parent relating 'to the ghost who is interposed – like a screen – between themselves and the child' (p 139). They give as an example the experiences of one mother who sought help for her baby boy, who had vomited feeds from birth. In the course of clinical consultation, the mother described the recent death of her brother, who also regurgitated (he had intestinal cancer). The connection made by the clinician ('he regurgitates like your brother') enabled the mother to separate her grief for her brother from her anxiety about her (boy) child. The clear and striking example of this 'ghost in the nursery' provides dramatic clinical possibilities. However, it also simplifies a complex configuration, in which it is as important to ask, as Reid implies in the example above, how the events remain so unmodified, despite time and experience.

Particularly in her discussion of infants who fail to thrive, Daws carefully elucidates the crucial experiences which influence parents and lead to feeding difficulties. Daws presents examples from her own work, which she connects with the work of Fraiberg. These examples all present a painful and distressing picture in which the withholding of food is usually supported by a parental rationalisation.

One example which Daws (1997) gives is of a three-week-old baby who was removed from home by workers after gaining no weight from birth. On reflection, it appeared that the older sister's jealousy was placated in that way – so that she, the sister, did not have to know that she had been displaced as the baby in the family.

This is, of course, a similar and probably more extreme example of the problems faced by Hester, whom I have described above. Some very powerful emotions were mobilised in the workers so that they too did not think about the new baby's needs. The rationalisation in this case was that the baby was not putting on weight, and fears of the infant's death were transmitted rather than thought about.

The painful sense of parental cruelty stems from the inability of parents (and workers) to notice and recognise the infant's needs, because of their own unmet needs, their inability to respond to the infant's needs, or feeling that they do not wish to share what they have with the infant. Daws concludes that:

> The major cause of the kind of feeding that leads to a withholding of food from the infant is undoubtedly the experience by the parent of neglect, deprivation and hunger in all its meanings, in their own childhood (Daws 1997, p 197).

The withholding of food should be seen as an emotional issue played out on a physical level. Unmet needs, 'ghosts in the nursery', and the legacy of deprived and disturbing experiences all form the material for experiences which are projected into the infant or child. Gianna Williams (1997), in her studies of infants, children and teenagers who have been subject to parental projection, discusses how the container–contained relationship is reversed through the parental expulsion of undigested experiences. Thus the child becomes a receptacle for these projections. In my own study (Briggs 1997), I observed how parental projections formed a particular and identifiable kind of parental interaction with infants. I called this 'convex containing shape'. The parent in these moments actively intrudes upon the infant. These intrusions can be primarily emotional intrusions of the parent's own uncontained, distressing or disturbing experiences, or they can be physical intrusions. They impact on the infant in a way which precipitates an 'at risk' situation for the infant, and, through repetition, affect a range of aspects of development.

Poor feeders

I have argued that parental deprivation, unmediated by past or current supportive relationships, has a central part to play in the development of feeding difficulties in infancy. However, it is also important within the parent–infant configuration to take into account the particular qualities the infant brings to the development of such difficulties or, alternatively, a capacity to overcome these difficulties. By this I mean that there is always a 'fit' between a mother and her infant. The degree of 'fit' depends not only on the mother's capacity in general, but also her particular capacity to deal with and respond to the constellation of feelings that are aroused in her by the baby. Some infants arouse in the mother a sense of her ability to understand and meet the needs of a particular baby. Feeding, at a physical and emotional level, is experienced as rewarding. On the other hand, some infants seem to push the mother beyond her own limitations or to arouse in her emotional experiences which are difficult for her.

Williams (1997) gives a striking example of a 'poor feeder'. This infant, whom she calls Robert, is from the beginning almost impossible to feed. He does not demand to be fed, when he is fed he regurgitates and instead sucks his thumb, his tongue and his lip. At two days old he:

> Made little stretching movements and his forehead was creased in a
> deep frown, a deep cleft on the lower lip was pulled up towards his
> mouth as though he was sucking in the flesh. Then he started to cry
> hard. His tongue was a little crescent raised inside his mouth (p 91).

The refusal of this infant to feed almost from the start of life aroused in the
mother a very disheartened state of mind. The more disheartened the mother
became, the less she felt she could meet his needs. This 'fit' between them –
perhaps more succinctly called a 'mis-fit' – led quickly to the development of a
pattern in which the infant's use of parts of the body, his hand, lip and tongue,
began to substitute for, or defend against, relying on another person to provide
him with what he needs. Eventually he needed to be tube-fed.

Some groups of infants are known to be poor feeders, including premature
babies (McFadyen 1994). Skuse (1993) emphasises the 'subtle interaction
between infant characteristics and parental response'. He distinguishes
between two groups of poor feeders – those who are restless, cry excessively
and do not complete feeds, and those who do not demand to be fed and go long
periods between feeds. The development of these difficulties can be related to
the qualities of the parent–infant relationship and, in particular, the qualities
of containment in the relationship. Problems in the capacity of the parent to
feed and of the infant to internalise the feed, at a physical and emotional level,
lead to infants relating in ways which express a lack of internalisation of good
experiences or which defend against the difficulties of depending on another
person.

The two patterns of infant feeding characteristics described by Skuse relate
closely to the relationship patterns demonstrated by infants in my study. The
first was a vigorously muscular kind of development, in which infants attempt
to use their bodies to achieve mastery over distress. These are the distressed,
restless feeders. One example is an infant, Timothy, whose mother feels she
does not have enough to offer him, and they become involved in a cycle of
distress, in which the mother feels she cannot understand or 'know what he
wants'. For example, at five months Timothy does not allow mother to be
separate from him:

> Timothy continued crying and mother said she was sewing. She went
> to him and gave him a mirror and a rattle. He looked round,
> continued to cry and then lifted himself up, leaning towards
> mother. He went right forward almost on to all fours and cried again.

Timothy shows by his movements that he wishes to be with his mother, and
that as she does not come towards him, he must move towards her. He did
reach physical milestones early, almost precociously. The mother seemed to
feel that he should be able to allow this degree of separation from her. This is
perhaps understandable at his age (five months), but the experiences of lack of

containment do not equip him, internally, to cooperate with this maternal wish.

The second pattern of relating was that infants withdrew from relationships in the face of either parental projections or unresponsiveness. These infants show a lack of emotional contact with others, lack of curiosity and a lack of evidence of physical development. Withdrawal from the world of relationships is accompanied by a closing down of attempts to make demands for attention and feeds. These infants also succeed in arousing considerable anxiety in others, particularly of a life and death dimension

Michael was one such infant. In the early weeks of life he demonstrated through his sucking gestures and his crying a wish to relate, feed and make demands. His withdrawal was dramatically worrying to observe. At times I watched him lie quietly with only the faintest signs of life and liveliness. For example, at three months:

> Michael was lying on his back with his eyes open the slightest amount. His mouth was open making some sucking movements. He lay still and moved his feet, turned his head slowly, still with his eyes open the merest crack.

He was sick in almost every feed I observed and at times he regurgitated almost the entire feed. His mother fed him irregularly and reluctantly. When she did feed him, she was intrusive and mechanical:

> Michael sucked at the bottle which Mary pushed backwards and forwards in and out of his mouth in a mechanical way, with impatience.

Similarly she was intrusive, and hostile, when wiping his mouth:

> Michael was sick and Mary vigorously mopped the corner of his mouth and his neck with tissue. He cried while she rubbed and stopped crying when she finished. He was sick again, and when Mary rubbed his mouth vigorously he cried.

On occasions, even as he appears most withdrawn, he could find it in him to respond to others, to become alert for a time and, almost covertly, to make developmental progress. There was a 'fit' between a mother who, through her antagonism towards him, wished her baby not to be there and a baby who made himself invisible. Failure to thrive physically was matched by difficulties in emotional development.

Infants like Michael demonstrate capacities and wishes to make contact, to feed and to demand feeding at birth and soon after. The pattern of withdrawal and muscularity clearly emerges as part of the process of the effects of the early relationship upon them. Developmental difficulties that are likely to be experienced by these infants are, first, as the example of Timothy shows, that they will have difficulty contending with experiences of separation. Weaning in particular may well be experienced as an unbearable loss or as a broken link with the mother.

Second, infants may develop difficulties in maintaining a relationship in which there is a trusting reliance or dependency on the parent. Not only does this affect what can be taken in at a physical level, but food itself can be rejected and/or felt to be contaminating. At an emotional level there is a parallel process in which learning can become impaired (Briggs 1995). In the case of Robert, discussed above, Williams makes an analogy between taking in food and taking in knowledge. It is clear that she is using this analogy as a metaphor, but, especially influenced by Bion's theories of thinking (1967), there is strong clinical evidence from work with children to suggest that feeding, internalising physical nourishment and love, is akin to internalising knowledge through thinking. Food for thought is a common expression which underscores this link. Daws points out that there is a connection between feeding difficulties and speech delays. The way these learning difficulties are seen in observational study is through difficulties in developing symbolic forms of communication. The following examples illustrate current psychoanalytic applications to children and young people with feeding difficulties and eating disorders (*see* Williams and Ravenscroft 1998).

Both Timothy and Michael, the infants described above, had difficulties with language development and symbolising in their play. Michael, in his play, demonstrated a close similarity between the quality of contact he had with his mouth on the teat and the difficulty he had in maintaining contact with an object when playing. His mouth became slack, loose and open; he had difficulty maintaining a grip on an object with his mouth. In his play, he also showed a difficulty in making a firm contact. For example, he played with a football when he was 14 months:

> He held it, pushed it, and he followed it; every contact pushing it away. He seemed to slip against it, with movements that were indecisive, neither trying to hold it nor move it.

His contact with the ball is very like his loose, open-mouthed contact with the bottle. Learning is difficult when there is such a loose grip on objects and relationships.

Timothy developed a mild food faddishness, which is clearly related to his feelings about father. At 20 months:

> Mother passed him his plate and said it was daddy's courgettes and tomatoes. Timothy took one mouthful and then made a face of distaste and spat out the food. Sally used a spoon to give him a mouthful. He took a fork and took a mouthful from this. Sally tried to sort out what he liked and what he did not, and then she said 'you

> really don't like it', adding to me that he usually ate most things. She gave him an apple and he began to eat it. Then he started to choke.

Disgust about father's 'courgettes and tomatoes' was probably connected with his reaction to recent events in the family, in which a second baby was conceived and miscarried. The attitude of disgust shows also a disturbance of trust and a problem in symbolising, in which the food is experienced concretely as parts of daddy's body. It is the concreteness of experience and the disturbance to the dependent relationship which forms the indigestible experience.

The evidence from regular, longitudinal observational studies of infants helps to substantiate the important connection between feeding difficulties, which emerge in the context of difficulties in the container–contained relationship, and the development of capacities to relate, to learn and to symbolise.

Summary

It has been shown that psychoanalytic theory, as exemplified by the work of object relations theorists such as Bion, Winnicott and Bick, underpins descriptions of parent–infant relationships in which emotionality is central to understanding the whole relationship. In this chapter, the emphasis has been placed on the impact on the early relationship between parents and infants of the parents' heightened emotionality and the intensity of early infantile experiences. In this early relationship, patterns of relating and fields of emotionality are laid down, and these are influential for future development. In Bion's theory of the container–contained relationship, the parent's role is to receive the intense communications from the infant and to respond sensitively and intuitively to the infant's communications, through 'reverie'. The quality of relating and the means for transforming emotions are essential parts of this theory. The feeding relationship is thought of as not simply concerning the physical processes – providing and taking in of food – but also as central to the processes of developing capacities to relate and share emotional states. The experience of feeding is therefore concerned with the development of the capacity to relate, to be intimate, to love, to hate and to think.

Difficulties in feeding emerge when there are problems in the relationship between 'container' and 'contained'. In this chapter, examples from clinical practice and observation have been used to describe the various ways in which feeding difficulties develop and how these may be connected with the particular difficulties both parents and infants bring to their feeding relationship. Parental deprivation, difficulties infants have of 'taking in', fear of separation and separateness, fear of intimacy, 'misfits' in the communication of emotions between parent and infant all have particular and distinctive implications for the feeding relationship. Examples have been given from a number of writers – among them Daws, Williams and my own studies – to illustrate and demonstrate themes that emerge in the parent–infant relationship where there are different kinds of feeding difficulties. These themes include problems that the parents transmit to the infant and their parenting role, through the parents' own earlier experiences, traumas, losses and deprivations; anxieties about separation and about intimacy; defending against infant vulnerability and missing the infant's communications, particularly those which seem to indicate a wish to relate and express emotionality; parental lack of confidence or anxieties aroused by the experience of previous babies, conscious or unconscious 'ghosts in the nursery' and projections into the infant of 'undigested' parental experience. These problems, which largely emanate from parental experiences, must also be seen alongside the differing individual characteristics infants bring to the feeding relationship. Examples of 'poor feeders' have been given to demonstrate problems parents may face in establishing a satisfactory feeding relationship, and how poor feeding may develop as a result of difficulty in the parent–infant relationship. Infants may then be seen as either becoming quite 'muscular' or withdrawing. It is important to differentiate the kind of dynamics which prevail in any parent–infant relationship in order to understand the qualities of the emotional life of both parent and infant which are impacting upon the problems in the feeding relationship.

In each early parent–infant relationship, distinctive patterns of relating emerge and these play a part in, and are influenced and transformed by, later experiences. Both the continuities in development and the changes, towards greater or less feeding difficulty, are influenced by the early configuration. The particular kind of feeding difficulty which can be observed – failure to take in, 'snack feeding', regurgitation of feeds and, in more extreme cases, failure to thrive – indicate particular patterns of difficulties in relating, and also to some extent predict the quality of difficulty which will be encountered in subsequent development. This chapter gives some illustrations of the kind of difficulties that may ensue in later development, especially those concerning difficulties with separation, in thinking and learning, and in symbolising and playing.

Professional intervention requires, first and foremost, detailed and repeated close observations of parent–infant relationships. The chapter has provided a discussion of the kind of observation training that is needed and has given examples from observations which illustrate the dynamics of feeding difficulties. Second, the professional needs to be able to understand the impact of the parent–infant relationship on himself or herself, not only through noting and thinking about how the work makes the worker feel, but what this might mean in terms of the parent–infant relationships. Appropriate professional intervention may then be guided by the sensitivity of these assessments and the worker's capacity to tolerate and think about anxieties that the parent–infant relationship cannot itself contain.

Conclusion

This chapter has discussed psychoanalytically based approaches to feeding difficulties, concentrating on the development of feeding relationships in infancy. Central to this approach are two fundamental ideas. First, that the dynamics of feeding relationships include a complex configuration of the parent–infant/child interactions and the internal worlds of parent and infant, which is constructed from current and past relationships. It follows that professional intervention when there are feeding difficulties needs to take account of all aspects of the dynamics of these relationships. Second, the process of infant feeding is synonymous with the development of relatedness; the experience of feeding means developing experiences of intimacy, separation and loss. The impact of feeding difficulties is inextricably connected to the emotionality of the parent–infant/child relationship.

Through observation and clinical encounters, a picture is built in which the impact of feeding difficulties on development can be associated closely with difficulties in thinking and learning. These insights into the impact of the dynamics in what Bion called the container–contained relationship have implications for professional practice based on thinking about the complex dynamics in parent–infant/child relationships.

References

Alvarez A (1992) *Live Company: psychoanalytic psychotherapy with autistic, border-line, deprived and abused children*. Routledge, London.

Bick E (1964) Notes on infant observation in psychoanalytic training. *International Journal of Psychoanalysis*. **45**: 484–8.

Bick E (1986) Further consideration of the function of the skin in early object relations: findings from infant observation integrated into child and adult analysis. *British Journal of Psychotherapy*. **2**(4): 292–301.

Bion W (1962) *Learning from Experience*. Heinemann, London.

Bion W (1967) *Second Thoughts*. Maresfield, London.

Brazelton T and Cramer B (1991) *The Earliest Relationship*. Karnac, London.

Briggs S (1992) Child observation and social work training. *Journal of Social Work Practice.* **6**(1): 49–61.

Briggs S (1995) Parallel process: emotional and physical digestion in adolescents with eating disorders. *Journal of Social Work Practice.* **9**(2): 155–68.

Briggs S (1997) *Growth and Risk in Infancy.* Jessica Kingsley, London.

Daws D (1993) Feeding problems and relationship difficulties: therapeutic work with parents and infants. *Journal of Child Psychotherapy.* **19**(2): 69–84.

Daws D (1995) Consultation in general practice. In: J Trowell and M Bower (eds) *The Emotional Needs of Young Children and Their Families.* Routledge, London.

Daws D (1997) The perils of intimacy: closeness and distance in feeding and weaning. *Journal of Child Psychotherapy.* **23**(2): 179–93.

Fraiberg S (1980) *Clinical Studies in Infant Mental Health.* Tavistock, London.

Harris M (1975) Notes on maternal containment in good enough mothering. Reprinted in M Harris Williams (ed) *The Collected Papers of Martha Harris and Esther Bick.* Clunie Press, Perthshire.

Klein M (1946) Notes on some schizoid mechanisms. Reprinted in Klein M (1988) *Envy and Gratitude and Other Works 1946–63.* Virago, London.

Klein M (1952) On observing the behaviour of young infants. Reprinted in Klein M (1988) *Envy and Gratitude and Other Works 1946–63.* Virago, London.

McFadyen A (1994) *Special Care Babies and their Developing Relationships.* Routledge, London.

Miller L *et al.* (eds) (1989) *Closely Observed Infants.* Duckworths, London.

Murray L (1992) The impact of postnatal depression on infant development. *Journal of Child Psychology and Psychiatry.* **33**(3): 543–61.

Piontelli A (1992) *From Fetus to Child.* Routledge, London.

Reid S (ed) (1997) *Developments in Infant Observation: the Tavistock Model.* Routledge, London.

Rustin M (1989) Reflections on method. In: L Miller *et al.* (eds) *Closely Observed Infants.* Duckworths, London.

Rustin M (1997) What do we see in the nursery? Infant observation as laboratory work. *International Journal of Infant Observation.* **1**(1): 93–110.

Skuse D (1993) Identification and management of problem eaters. *Archives of Diseases in Childhood.* **69**: 604–8.

Stern D (1985) *The Interpersonal World of the Infant.* Basic, New York.

Tanner K and Le Riche P (1998) *Observation and its Application to Social Work: rather like breathing.* Jessica Kingsley, London.

Williams G (1997) *Internal Landscapes and Foreign Bodies.* Duckworths, London.

Williams G and Ravenscroft K (1998) *Feeding Difficulties in Childhood and Eating Disorders in Adolescence.* Jason Aronson, Washington.

Winnicott D (1964) *The Child, the Family and the Outside World.* Penguin, Harmondsworth.

Winnicott D (1965) *The Maturational Processes and the Facilitating Environment.* Hogarth, London.

Winnicott D (1974) Fear of breakdown. *International Review of Psychoanalysis.* **1**(1): 103–7.

Further reading

Brazelton T, Koslowski B and Main M (1974) The origins of reciprocity: the early mother–infant interaction. In: M Lewis and L Rosenblum (eds) *The Effect of the Infant on its Caregiver.* Wiley, New York.

Menzies Lyth I (1988) *Containing Anxiety in Institutions.* Free Association Books, London.

Obholzer A and Roberts V (1994) *The Unconscious at Work.* Routledge, London.

CHAPTER 5

Developmental, regulatory and cognitive aspects of feeding disorders

Gillian Harris

Introduction

There has been a long history in interventions carried out with children who fail to thrive of 'mother blaming'; that is, assuming that the problem in the child is caused by the nature of the relationship between child and mother. Indeed, some of the research studies carried out appear to give support to the idea that a failure to gain weight in the child is related to the attachment status with the mother (Gordon and Jameson 1970). However, these studies quite often do not have appropriate control groups, nor do they address the problem that the difficulty in feeding a child may affect the way a mother feels about her child, and that this in turn may manifest in behaviour which leads to an insecure attachment classification. Alternatively, there may be something about the temperament of the child which contributes both to the feeding problem and to the behaviour which defines the attachment criteria. Lindberg *et al.* (1994), in a longitudinal study of infants with failure to thrive, identified 'difficultness' of temperament as one of the defining characteristics of the infants they were assessing. It is possible, therefore, to move from a model of feeding problems which concentrates primarily on the relationship with the mother or care-giver to one which incorporates difficulties that the child may bring to the feeding interaction. Before we do this, however, the nature of the feeding problem itself should be defined.

Defining the problem

There are two forms of behaviour that parents and professionals may describe as a feeding problem; these may occur together or separately in any one child.

The first 'behaviour' is that of a refusal by the child to take sufficient calories to enable the expected growth velocity. The second is a refusal to take in a sufficiently wide range of foods to constitute a balanced diet. There are, of course, subjective components to both of these stated problems. First, the concept of 'sufficient' calories is a difficult one, since children with different metabolic rates could eat widely varying amounts of food and still grow along the same trajectory. The decision about whether or not a child takes sufficient calories can, therefore, only really be made on whether or not the child is growing appropriately. If the child is not growing at all then this assumption cannot be questioned. However, if the child is growing, but slowly, there may still be problems. The 'expected' growth trajectory may not be appropriate for the child; that is, parents or professionals may expect the child to be heavier or to grow taller than they are genetically determined to do. We also have to remember that decisions about the appropriateness of growth cannot be made on a single 'height' or 'weight' in isolation. The child's weight needs to be assessed in relation to height, and we would need a number of heights and weights collected over time to fully understand the child's pattern of growth so we might relate this understanding to the child's observed feeding 'problem'. Second, there are difficulties in defining a 'balanced diet', for what is thought to constitute a balanced diet differs from person to person, from decade to decade, and from culture to culture.

The second problem behaviour, that of refusing to take a suffcient range of foods, may therefore also be confounded by the subjective nature of diagnosis, although this difficulty may be slightly ameliorated if the problem is considered in terms of its severity. A refusal to take sufficient foods can either be relatively common food fussiness or the less common problem of food perseveration. Food fussiness we may define as a refusal to take on one day a food which has been accepted on another day. Food perseveration, however, is a rigid adherence to specific foods, with a marked fear of unknown or disliked foods.

Once the nature of the feeding problem and its relation to growth has been established, bearing in mind that a child may be both failing to grow appropriately (failing to thrive) and showing perseverant eating tendencies, then the contribution that the child may make to the 'observed' feeding problem can be determined.

Children who present in a feeding clinic with either form of food refusal are only very rarely best described as 'being naughty'; that is, the parent is not as good at child management as the child is at parent management. There is usually a reason for the child's behaviour, which lies either in the child's developmental history, specifically that pertaining to the acquisition of food preferences and experiences, or in the child's ability to self-regulate.

The development of food preferences

Infants are born with a clear preference for a sweet taste (Desor *et al.* 1975); the response shown to the other tastes is less clear-cut. The infant's response to a salt taste has been described as both neutral and aversive according to the methodology used in the specific study (Crook 1978). We would not expect a salt taste to be markedly aversive, however, because the neonate has experienced the taste of salt, at a low level, in amniotic fluid. Similarly, the neonate finds a sour taste both interesting and slightly unpleasant (Johnson and Harris 1998). The taste which produces the clearest aversion is bitter; the neonate will show a facial expression which is indicative of pain in response to a bitter taste (Johnson and Harris 1998). Neonates also find the 'taste' of water aversive. The function of these preferences and aversions is of course to direct the neonate into taking a high-calorie, sweet fluid, such as breast milk, rather than water, which has no energy value, or bitter, highly salt and sour fluids which may well be toxic. The tastes of salt, sour and bitter cannot, however, remain aversive to the infant as he or she grows older, or the adult diet would be dominated by sweet-tasting food. The infant has, during the weaning period, to learn to like all the different tastes, not in fluids, but in foods.

There is no evidence to show that humans are able to selectively eat different foods to provide us with specific elements of the diet in which we may be deficient. The exception to this is salt: those who are salt depleted crave salt (Beauchamp 1987). We cannot then expect children to eat a 'balanced' diet by instinct. All of our food preferences are a function of exposure (Pliner 1982); we learn to like those foods we have eaten, and we eat those foods we have learned to like. Infants have therefore to learn to like the foods that are safe and culturally appropriate for them to eat. This learning is achieved during the weaning process.

Weaning foods are usually offered to infants from the age of approximately 14 weeks, at an age when milk can no longer be taken in sufficient amounts to meet energy requirements (Harris 1988). From this age, through to about six months, the infant is unusually receptive to new tastes. In fact, this period might be thought of as a developmental window of acceptance (Harris *et al.* 1990). During this period, parents offer the infant the foods they consider to be both culturally acceptable and safe. When offered such new foods, with all but those of a sweet taste, the infant may show a facial expression which indicates some initial distaste. However, for all but the most bitter-tasting foods (such as foods in the cabbage family), with repeated exposure the infant rapidly learns to like the taste of the foods that have been given (Harris 1993b). By the end of the first year of life these learned taste preferences develop into very clear food preferences. The infant shows a preference for the foods that have been given and these preferences are very specific (Harris and Booth 1987). The infant's preference for a food will be for a known recipe; that is, a 'gestalt' of taste, texture and context. This is why infants, at this age, are very difficult to wean from commercial baby food recipes to home-prepared versions. Commercial baby foods have standard recipes (tastes and textures), which will be very different from a home-prepared version.

This development of taste and food preferences occurs along with the development of the skills necessary to suck, sip and chew. It is well known that neonates must have experience of sucking in the early weeks if they are not to lose the sucking reflex, and so those infants who are not able to ingest foods are usually given the appropriate experience of sucking. It is less well recognised that there may be a similar sensitive period for the ability to cope with foods of firmer texture; that is, foods which have to be moved around the mouth and chewed rather than swallowed 'whole' (Monahan *et al.* 1988). In the first year, therefore, an infant may miss out on sensitive periods which relate to both taste and food preferences as well as to oromotor function. Clinically, such children with adverse early feeding histories may present with a dependence on either a limited range of foods or a limited range of textures (Harris and Booth 1992). The foods most usually depended upon are those that have been given as 'baby' foods, such as sweet custard or commercially prepared foods. Similarly, the child may present with a dependence on milk, whether breast- or bottle-fed. A child who has missed out on the period in which textured foods should be introduced, from nine to 15 months, may surprisingly present with a 'behavioural' feeding problem; that is, as a 'naughty' child. Both parents, and others from the medical professions, often have difficulty understanding why it is that a child can eat crisps but can't eat meat and will insist on eating only yoghurts that are lump-free. It is, of course, important to remember that children with secondary oromotor dysfunction may have this problem as a result of more general problems with motor coordination (Wolf and Glass 1992): not all children who can't chew have missed out on a sensitive period.

Regulatory function

Although it has not been shown that children and adults are able to regulate their diets to achieve a balance of nutrients, it has been shown that both children and adults can regulate their diets to achieve an appropriate calorie load (Keesey 1978). In adults, this means that when we are not attempting to lose weight by 'dieting', we tend to take a constant calorie load to accord with energy output and maintain a stable weight. In children, it is more complex. Children have to take in an appropriate calorie load which both accords with energy output and enables growth on the determined trajectory. This ability can be seen in infants as young as six weeks, at which age it has been demonstrated that infants fed formulae with calorie densities different from the milk formula usually fed to them adjusted their intake accordingly (Fomon *et al.* 1969, 1976). The infants were not able to make absolute adjustments in calorie intake, but they did take more or less calories depending on whether the new formula was more or less calorie-dense than the one normally fed to them. This ability to regulate calorie intake becomes more exact as the infant develops and, by the age of four years, children allowed to choose their own food over a period of time will take in a constant number of calories (Birch and Deysher 1986). The number of calories taken by a child or by an adult may, however, vary on a day-to-day basis or even on a week-to-week basis. That is, children may well have good and bad days, and only if you compare the calorie intake for a whole week with that of the next week will regulation be observed. As many illnesses interfere with appetite, where the child has had some form of intercurrent infection, regulation may only be observed in month-to-month comparisons (Harris and Booth 1992). The child will stop eating during a period of ill health and weight will either stabilise or drop. However, in a child who is able to regulate, compensatory eating will occur when the period of illness has passed. Usually this process of compensation is not noticed by parent or carer.

In a normally well child, weight is not consistently monitored, and small fluctuations pass unnoticed. In a child with a 'good' appetite and growth, days of not eating are not a source of anxiety. In the child with a chronic illness or with 'poor' appetite and growth, however, days of not eating are not accepted with equanimity. Parents of children of 'poor' appetite are likely to perceive periods of not eating not as part of the regulatory cycle, but as indicative of a general decline in appetite, and will initiate a period of coercive or forceful feeding. It has frequently been observed that maladaptive feeding interactions between parent and child are often a response to anxiety on the part of the parent about poor growth or feeding on the part of the child. This anxiety may be in response to health concerns about the child. Anxiety-related forceful feeding is often observed in parents of children who have illnesses such as cystic fibrosis, where the life expectancy of the child is dependent on good nutritional status (Harris and MacDonald 1992) and is also observed where parents have a child who is growth compromised, such as children with Silver Russell syndrome (Blisset 1998).

Parents of children who have a growth disorder, as well as parents of children who are just short in stature, are not always aware that the child's intake is determined by growth potential; that is, that intake is regulated to accord with growth. Such parents tend to think that intake determines growth, that there is no genetic or physiological limiter. Of course, if sufficient calories are not made available to a child then growth will be compromised, but more than sufficient calories will not enable additional growth. For some children it also seems to be clear that this regulatory ability is impaired in a way that is not yet fully understood. In any sample of children with failure to thrive, there seems always to be a subgroup who are smaller than would be expected from family heights and yet have no organic problems to explain this disparity. The child's weight does not falter, but rather follows along its own trajectory, usually around the 0.4th centile. These children are often weight-for-height appropriate, active, bright and well cared for but seemingly without appetite. As infants, such children have been reported as sleeping through feeds if not woken, without crying (Skuse *et al.* 1992). Such children may be thought of as having poor regulatory function, and do not show good compensatory feeding.

Regulation and supplementation

Regulatory function also needs to be taken into consideration when assessing the appetite for 'solid' food in children who gain their calories from another source. Children who are still mainly dependent on breast- or bottle-feeding after the first year are difficult to wean on to solid foods, not only because they have missed the developmental window of acceptance (Illingworth and Lister 1964) but also because their calorie needs are met by the milk. They have no 'motivation' to move on to a different calorie source. This is especially true of children with oromotor dysfunction, who may have learnt from past experience to find solid food aversive. Similarly, children who are given calorie supplements to aid weight gain, or who are tube-fed, will show compensation (Harris 1993a). Normal eating behaviour may well occur alongside the supplemental feeding for some weeks, but then oral feeding will decline. In children who are maintained, perhaps from necessity, on high-calorie loads via a tube-feed, all normal feeding may disappear until the milk load can be decreased (Warady *et al.* 1990). Where young children have to be tube-fed in order to maintain or develop oral feeding, the strategy to aim for is to encourage the 'experience' of feeding. That is, very small amounts of different tastes and textures should be encouraged during the sensitive periods. These foods should be fed at the time of day when the child is most hungry (the evening for an overnight tube-fed child), rather than an attempt being made to feed 'normal' meals.

Learning about calories

Regulation of calorie intake is of course mediated by learning and this learning fits into the developmental agenda. Children have to 'learn' the calorie load of each food in order that they might regulate their intake, although this learning does not occur at a conscious level (Logue 1991). The learned association between food and the calorific consequences of ingestion is dependent on an association being made between the taste of the food and its calorie load. This is made easier if a food is eaten more than once, and much of the regulation of eating is a regulation of meal times. We become hungry at certain times for the calorie load that we usually have at that particular time. So in order to be hungry for breakfast at 9 am, we have to have had breakfast at 9 am on preceding days. If we miss out a regular meal, then we will compensate by eating more later. If we continue to miss out the meal then we will stop feeling hungry at that time. This learnt meal-time hunger is the rationale behind the intervention strategy used with children of poor or small appetite who do not seem to regulate well (Harris 1994). The way to optimise intake is to feed small meals frequently, rather than leave the child to get hungry. A poorly regulating child left to get hungry will eat less than a poorly regulating child who is fed at two-hourly intervals. A child who regulates well will of course be able to maintain their intake even with long periods of time between meals.

Perseverance and cognitive development

The 'flattening' out of growth after the first year, a decline in growth velocity which is accompanied by a decline in the rate of increase of appetite, is a time at which many children start to be seen as 'fussy' or 'picky' by their parents (Williamson *et al.* 1998). Also at this age, as the child develops in need for autonomy, the sudden refusal of a food that was once eaten is likely to occur. This is 'normal' fussiness. So, too, is the refusal to eat a food that has never been tasted on the grounds that the child 'wouldn't like it' (Birch and Marlin 1982). This response shows the increasing onset of neophobia (Pliner and Loewen 1997), the refusal to try new foods, which starts to develop during the first year. The neophobic response probably has evolutionary advantage. A potential food that has not been introduced in the early months as appropriate and safe may well turn out to be poisonous. In later childhood years, new foods are usually only tried if others are seen to eat them first (Harper and Sanders 1985); imitation dissipates neophobia. Foods that children have eaten and learned to include in their repertoire are possibly categorised according to perceptual cues, first taste and smell, then by the way foods look (Morgan and Greene 1994). Anything that doesn't fit into these early categories will be rejected, quite literally on sight (Birch 1993). Later foods may be accepted, or at least tried, if they belong to a known conceptual category, mediated by language: 'it may look unusual but because I am told it is a biscuit and I like biscuits I will try it'. Although these rejections of new foods are universal, there do seem to be differences in the extent to which both adults and children are likely to try new foods. This difference in willingness to try foods varies according to temperament (Pliner and Loewen 1997). Very neophobic children score high on emotionality scales and low on sociability scales of standardised measures of temperament. A low sociability score denotes a child who is unlikely to be influenced by the actions of others. Therefore a very neophobic child will be less likely to copy others and eat new foods that they observe others eating.

Children may therefore be seen to eat only a narrow range of foods for two reasons. First, a wide range of foods has not been introduced early enough before the onset of neophobia. Second, the child may be temperamentally disinclined to try new foods after the onset of neophobia.

By the age of four years the neophobic response seems to be well established, and the conceptual categories of food types that will be eaten and food types that will not be eaten are well developed. Clinical observation suggests that it becomes extremely difficult after this age to widen the range of foods eaten by young children. This is mainly because children between the ages of four and 14 years lack the motivation to widen the range of foods that they eat. Any presenting 'feeding problem' is, after all, usually the parents' 'problem', in that it is the parents' concern rather than the concern of the child. Teenagers may, however, gain motivation to change from peer-group pressure, and new foods can quite often be introduced at this later age.

Perseverant feeding disorder

Some children who eat only a very narrow range of foods, perhaps as few as four or five foods, and who rigidly adhere to this diet may just have extreme forms of 'temperamental' neophobia. However, extremely neophobic children seem to be truly perseverant and adhere rigidly to preferences not only for specific foods, but also to particular brands of certain foods and particular flavours within that brand of food. They also show an extreme fear response if they are asked to try new foods and a contamination response if a liked food touches an unliked food. This fear and contamination response is, however, the extreme form of the universal disgust response (Rozin 1986). Those foods that are not part of our known repertoire do, to a greater or lesser extent, become disgusting to us. Further, a food that is not part of our repertoire might well 'contaminate' an accepted food, were the two to touch. So we could say that children with a perseverant feeding problem are at the extreme end of a normal continuum. However, many children with autism and Asperger's syndrome show perseverant feeding disorder, and those children who present with the disorder but who are not within the autistic spectrum tend to be boys. The feeding style of these children often seems to change in their second year from 'good eaters' to 'fussy eaters'. As a group, the children tend to be more anxious and more fearful of new stimuli. However, those children who do not fulfil the criteria for autism or Asperger's syndrome but are perseverant in feeding style have good social skills and do not have mentalising problems. It may well be that this group of children have problems in the transition from the perceptual distinction between foods (that is, the way they smell, taste or look) to the general conceptual categories of foods. Often children with perseverant feeding disorder will smell foods before they eat them or adhere to food of only one colour. Therefore, because there is no generalisation to conceptual category, each new flavour and each different brand (which will of course have a slightly different smell, taste and look) evokes the neophobic response. A dysfunction in the ability to generalise would explain the rigidity of preference, the contamination fears and the extreme neophobic responses seen in children who present with perseverant feeding disorders. Regulatory function in such children is intact; if children with a perseverant feeding disorder are allowed to eat the foods they like, then weight gain and growth are not compromised.

In young children with perseverant feeding disorder, the range of foods eaten can only be increased gradually. The child should be allowed to eat mainly the foods that they like; new foods should be introduced gradually and without coercion. Some children will agree to taste new foods, although others may refuse to put an unknown food in their mouth. Those that do agree to taste foods should be allowed first to choose which foods they will taste, and then to choose which of the tasted foods they will try to include in their diet. A new food should be offered in extremely small portions a few times a week until a point of acceptance has been reached. The new food needs then to be maintained in the child's diet, but at first still in small portions. Children who will not taste new foods may be encouraged to try slightly different foods to those that they already like, such as a different flavour of crisp or a different type of biscuit. The aim of this approach is to help the child make the category generalisations that they have hitherto failed to make. Occasionally, children with this type of feeding problem will eat an entirely new food in a new context when they see others eating. This, however, is a rare event. Perseverant eaters do not usually show a general increase in the range of foods accepted if they sit with other adults or with other children at, for example, a school meal time. Nor does playing with food or helping to prepare foods increase their dietary range, although it may help to reduce the neophobic response to the foods by desensitising the child to specific food smells.

Conclusion

It can be seen that there are two dimensions to feeding behaviour in children: regulatory function and the extent of the neophobic response. These two dimensions map roughly on to the two presentations of feeding problems in children, namely those of not taking sufficient calories or not taking a sufficiently wide range of foods. Both dimensions are affected by the developmental agenda, which determines when and how hunger is expressed. Both dimensions, and the learned component of appetite, interact in turn with the feeding management style of the parent. Whether the problem is one of too little food eaten or of too few foods eaten, the intervention should start at the same point – that of returning control of eating to the child. The child should be given small, frequent meals of food they like, without regard to dietary balance. Wherever possible the child should be moved on from spoon feeding to self-feeding. In addition, when implementing these programmes, it is of paramount importance that the parent should be closely supported, in order that parental anxiety about child intake can be carefully managed.

References

Beauchamp GK (1987) The human preference for excess salt. *American Scientist.* **75**: 27–32.

Birch LL (1993) Children, parents and food. *British Journal of Food.* **95**(9): 11–16.

Birch LL and Deysher M (1986) Caloric compensation and sensory specific satiety: evidence of self-regulation of food intake by young children. *Appetite.* **7**: 323–31.

Birch LL and Marlin DW (1982) I don't like it, I never tried it: effects of exposure to food on two-year-old children's food preferences. *Appetite.* **3**: 353–60.

Blisset J (1998) Feeding problems in children with growth disorders. PhD thesis, University of Birmingham.

Crook CK (1978) Taste perception in the newborn infant. *Infant Behaviour and Development.* **1**: 52–69.

Desor JA, Mailer O and Andrews K (1975) Ingestive responses of human newborns to salty, sour and bitter stimuli. *Journal of Comparative and Physiological Psychology.* **89**(8): 966–70.

Fomon SJ, Filer LJ, Thomas LN, Anderson TA and Nelson SE (1969) Relationship between formula concentration and rate of growth of normal infants. *Journal of Nutrition.* **98**: 241–54.

Fomon SJ, Thomas LN, Filer LJ, Anderson TA and Nelson SE (1976) Influence of fat and carbohydrate content of diet on food intake and growth of male infants. *Acta Paediatrica Scandinavica.* **64**: 136–44.

Gordon AH and Jameson JC (1970) Infant–mother attachment in patients with non-organic failure to thrive syndrome. *Journal of the American Academy of Child Psychiatry.* **18**: 251–9.

Harper L and Sanders K (1985) The effects of adult eating on young children's acceptance of unfamiliar foods. *Journal of Experimental Child Psychology.* **20**: 206–14.

Harris G (1988) Determinants of the introduction of solid food. *Journal of Reproductive and Infant Psychology.* **6**: 241–9.

Harris G (1993a) Feeding problems and their treatment. In: I St James Roberts, G Harris and D Messer (eds) *Infant Crying, Feeding and Sleeping; development, problems and treatment.* Harvester Wheatsheaf, Herts.

Harris G (1993b) Introducing the infant's first solid food. *British Food Journal.* **95**(9): 7–10.

Harris G (1994). *QED: Food Fights.* London: BBC Education Developments.

Harris G and Booth DA (1987) Infants' preference for salt in food: its dependence upon recent dietary experience. *Journal of Reproductive and Infant Psychology.* **5**: 97–104.

Harris G and Booth IW (1992) The nature and management of eating problems in pre-school children. In: PJ Cooper and A Stein (eds) *Feeding Problems and Eating Disorders in Children and Adolescents*, pp. 61–84. Harwood Academic Publishers, Chur.

Harris G and MacDonald A (1992) Behavioural feeding problems in cystic fibrosis. *Paediatric Pulmonology* (Supplement 8). Wiley, New York.

Harris G, Thomas A and Booth DA (1990) Development of salt taste in infancy. *Developmental Psychology.* **26**(4): 534–8.

Illingworth RS and Lister J (1964) The critical or sensitive period with specific reference to certain feeding problems in infants and children. *Journal of Pediatrics.* **65**: 839–48.

Johnson R and Harris G (1998) Infant facial expression in response to gustatory stimuli of different qualities and intensities. ICIS, Atlanta, Georgia.

Keesey RE (1978) Set-points and body weight regulation. *Psychiatric Clinics of North America.* **1**: 523–43.

Lindberg L, Bohlin G, Hagekull B and Thunstrom M (1994) Early food refusal: infant and family characteristics. *Infant Mental Health Journal.* **15**(3): 262–77

Logue AW (1991) *The Psychology of Eating and Drinking.* Freeman, New York.

Monahan P, Shapiro B and Fox C (1988) Effect of tube-feeding on oral function. *Developmental Medicine and Child Neurology.* **57**(7): 12.

Morgan J and Greene T (1994) An analysis of categorization style in pre-schoolers. *Psychological Reports.* **74**: 59–66.

Pliner P (1982) The effects of mere exposure on liking for edible substances. *Appetite.* **3**: 353–60.

Pliner P and Loewen ER (1997) Temperament and food neophobia in children and their mothers. *Appetite.* **28**: 239–54.

Rozin P (1986) One trial acquired likes and dislikes in humans: disgust as a US, food predominance and negative learning predominance. *Learning and Motivation.* **17**: 180–9.

Skuse D, Wolke D and Reilly S (1992) Failure to thrive: clinical and developmental aspects. In: H Remschmidt and M Schmidt (eds) *Child and Youth Psychiatry:*

European Perspectives, vol II, *Developmental Psychopathology*. Hogrefe and Huber, Lewiston.

Warady BA, Kriely M, Belkden B, Hellerstein S and Man U (1990) Nutritional and behavioural aspects of nasogastric tube-feeding in infants receiving chronic peritoneal dialysis. *Advances in Peritoneal Dialysis*. **6**: 265–8.

Williamson D, Prether R, Heffer R and Kelley M (1988) Eating disorder: psychological therapies. In: JL Marston (ed) *Handbook of Treatment and Approaches in Childhood Psychopathology*. Plenum Press, New York.

Wolf L and Glass R (1992) *Feeding and Swallowing Disorders in Infancy*. Therapy Skill Builders, Tucson, Arizona.

Further reading

Peichat ML and Rozin P (1982) The special role of nausea in the acquisition of food dislikes by humans. *Appetite*. **3**: 341–51.

Rosenstein R and Oster H (1988) Differential facial responses to four basic tastes in newborns. *Child Development*. **59**: 1555–68.

CHAPTER 6

Cultural aspects of feeding: some illustrations from the Indian culture

Kedar Nath Dwivedi

Introduction

Culture influences virtually all aspects of human behaviour and practices and perhaps none more so than food and feeding habits. Although it would be extremely useful to compile a body of knowledge in this respect from many different cultures, such a compilation would be beyond both the scope of this chapter and the expertise of the current author. It is proposed therefore to exemplify the above with illustrations mainly from the Indian culture. The chapter looks at food and emotion, cultural rites, religious cosmology relating to food, and the impact of culture on social identity and child-rearing. It also covers the ascribed properties of food and ends by examining elements pertaining to the professional relationship within a multicultural setting.

In the past, it was assumed that living for long periods of time in different geographical environments led to different groups developing their characteristic inborn temperaments. Categorisation has moved through several stages, based on the philosophical climate and zeitgeist, culminating in beliefs which have shaped our understanding of different peoples.

In recent years, therefore, a 'new culture and personality' approach has emerged that aims to go beyond the 'old culture and personality' movement, which was essentially Eurocentric (Stocking 1986). The new approach attempts to understand cultures from their own indigenous ideological perspectives in order to conceptualise contrasting human nature. Geertz (1973), therefore, sees culture as a 'web of meaning' and Laungani (1992) emphasises the fact that 'It is these assumptions which often are culture-specific. Not the experience itself as has been mistakenly assumed by the cultural relativists' (p 223).

Just like individuals, cultures also grow and mature. In a multicultural context we have people and societies belonging to cultures that may be many millennia old living side by side with those belonging to cultures that are only a few centuries old. For example, in the Indian culture, as early as the 6th century BC, a detailed, coherent and systematic theory of consciousness became available, something that did not begin to happen in the Western science until the 19th century AD (Reat 1990).

Food and emotion

In the Indian culture, one finds a huge variety of paths to salvation (Dwivedi and Prasad 1999). These range from subjugating feelings and emotions through the rigours of asceticism (such as in Jainism and most schools of Buddhism and Hinduism) to encouraging exuberant emotional and sensuous experiences (such as in the Ajivika and Tantric schools in Hinduism and Buddhism) exemplified by the *Kamasutra*. For example, Ajivikas (8th century BC) challenged the karmic theory and gave the slogan 'eat, drink and be merry'. Pushti Marg (Bennett 1990) is an example of exciting the passions as a form of worship.

There can also be cultural differences in the very conceptualisation of emotions. The Western conceptualisation of emotion has had its emphasis on the physiological and irrational aspects of emotions. Recently, however, the social constructivists and cognitivists have begun to point out the fact that emotions are essentially culturally constructed appraisals. For example, Lynch (1990a) shows that:

> Contrary to Western devaluation of emotion in the face of reason, India finds emotions, like food, necessary for a reasonable life, and, like taste, cultivable for the fullest understanding of life's meaning and purpose. . . . (p 23).

In the Indian way of thinking, the mind and body are part of, and continuous with, one another and thus identical. Therefore, emotions are grounded not only in self but also in food, scent, music, play and so on. For example, an offering, such as food, is conceived as the embodiment of an emotional attitude (such as devotion to god): 'In offering the food to god, in its return to his devotee, and in its consumption as *prasada*, emotions are believed to be exchanged between humanity and divinity' (Lynch 1990b, p 103). Food left over from god is called *prasada* and its consumption by the devotee is to experience the self transformed through the act of giving. The proper equivalent of saying grace in the Indian culture is not so much of thanking god for the food, but offering food to god and then eating the leftovers.

In most cultures, life-cycle rites such as initiations and weddings are often used for the purposes of transformation. Bennett (1990) describes ritual as:

a culturally constructed system of symbolic communication comprising a structured sequence of words and acts directed towards a 'telic' or 'performative' outcome.

He continues:

Ritual has the capacity to shape and intensify experience by means of patterning, sequencing, repetition, and the controlled arrangement of multiple sensory media (Bennett 1990, p 185).

In the Indian culture, these rites (or *Sanskaras* in Sanskrit) are meant to have a refining quality (as evident from the meaning of this Sanskrit word) and this refining process has essentially three main phases: physical, mental and spiritual. As Marglin (1990) writes:

The process of refining implies that one starts with a concrete or physical or gross level and by successive processes of refinement extracts from these concrete emotions their essence. The basic processes of refining are cooking, and the most basic cooking is that which takes place in the earth when a seed germinates under the heat of the sun and the moisture of water. The grain or fruit that is eventually produced out of this cooking is the refined product. When the body is refined, out of its physicality several refined products emerge: emotions, thought and finally, the most refined product of all, corresponding to the fragrance of the food offered to the deities, spiritual experience (pp 231–2).

The Indian theory of 'Rasa'

The Indian theory of emotions known as the 'Rasa (essence, flavour, extract, juice) theory' was established several millennia ago, as evident in Bharat's famous Treatise on Natyashastra (dramatology) of 200 BC, outlining the catalytic purpose of aesthetic forms to activate and refine our already present emotions (de Bary *et al.* 1958; Dwivedi 1993b; Dwivedi and Gardner 1997).

In such a cultural context, food is perceived not only as containing nutrients but also emotion and morality and its purity is as important as (sometimes more important than) its nutrient value. Food is supposed to become easily impure while it is being prepared, as it is imbued with the moral and emotional qualities of those who prepare it. Thus, purity of thoughts, feelings, conduct and actions while preparing food is also very important. A food prepared and offered lovingly, selflessly and solely for the enjoyment of the eater is more likely to be pure. Thus, food is supposed not only to affect the moral and emotional disposition of the eater, but it can also be imbued and invested with the moral and emotional qualities of those who prepare and offer it (Bennett 1990). In this sense, it is therefore difficult to be sure of purity in ready-to-eat food obtained from supermarkets, restaurants, hospitals and so on.

There is no doubt that such cultural ideologies in their full form may not be operative in many Indians today, living in either India or in the West. However, these are often present at least in diluted forms and influence many practices around food, feeding and eating (e.g. bringing food into hospital). A professional's appreciation of this cultural dynamic is essential for a better sharing of concerns and strategies between the professionals and families.

Implications of the Indian theory of karma on vegetarianism and feeding

In the Indian culture, the attempt to make sense of the existential issues began as early as during the Indus Valley civilisation and continued through the Vedic period culminating in an elaborate cosmology by the Vedantic or Upanishadic period (Table 6.1). The Vedantic ideology is an amazing synthesis of the Yogic concept of individual soul from the Indus Valley civilisation and the cosmic concept of world soul (god) derived from the Vedic culture (Reat 1990). The individual soul is a reflection of the cosmic soul (as in the modern analogy of a hologram) and has a layered consciousness. It goes through the cycle of birth and rebirth in different planes of existence according to one's karma.

The karmic theory is a theory of cause and effect. It states that all volitional

Table 6.1: The historical aspect of ideological developments in India

Period	Ideological aspects
Indus Valley civilisation (5000 BC–2500 BC)	Yogic concepts of individual soul; layered consciousness; rebirth and release
Vedic period (2500 BC–1200 BC)	Cosmogonic concept of world soul; rituals; afterlife
Vedantic period (1200 BC–500 BC)	Upanishads linking the world soul with individual soul, layered consciousness, karma and rebirth
Heterodox schools (800 BC–200 AD)	Ajivikism; Jainism; Buddhism
Revival of Hinduism (200 AD onwards)	Buddhism, having spread abroad, deteriorated in India. Hinduism included revival of Vedic authority, Smrities, Yoga, Sankhya, Mimansa, Nyaya and Vedanta

actions lead to consequences, not in the sense of someone dishing out consequences but in the sense of seeds turning into fruits, given the right conditions and right amount of time. Volitional actions also include speech and thoughts with intention. Actions (karma) can be performed in a short time but their consequences can last for a very long time. Consequently, there may be a long backlog of karma that have been performed already and are still in the queue waiting to turn into consequences, perhaps for many lifetimes (Dwivedi and Prasad 1999).

All sentient beings are caught in this cycle of birth and rebirth in different planes of existence until they manage to free themselves through salvation, nirvana or enlightenment. One can be reborn in any plane of existence (e.g. god, human, animal, ghost and so on) depending upon one's actions or karma. Thus, a non-vegetarian food may come from an animal (i.e. a sentient being) that might have been one's parent, partner, sibling or offspring in a previous life. In addition, killing or being intentionally responsible for the killing of any sentient being can also have its negative karmic consequences.

It is understandable that in such an ideological climate, many Indians are vegetarian. However, they find that the strength of their feeling in this respect, in the Western context, is seldom fully appreciated. Many (at least during their early days of being in the West) also feel shocked by the abhorrent sight of animal carcasses hanging in the butchers' shops (Dwivedi R 1996). The sight of non-vegetarian food can arouse a similar feeling in some. The concept of purity mentioned above also influences their feelings towards consuming vegetarian food which may have been in contact with a non-vegetarian food, cooking utensils, equipment, site and so on.

One of the Buddhist and/or Hindu precepts for monks or nuns involves not taking anything unless it is given to them, such as not eating unless it has been served in their bowl. It is also traditional for Indian hosts to serve food on their guest's plate for the same reason. It prevents the guest from performing a negative karma (of taking what is not formally given) and allows the host to gain merits by giving. The same principle is extended to feeding the other with one's own fingers, particularly in a very loving relationship. Parents often do this to their young children as an expression of their love. Similarly, partners feed each other, as an essential part of the wedding ritual (Figure 6.1).

Cultural ideology, social structure and child-rearing

Child-rearing practices can differ widely across cultures depending upon their sociocultural and ideological differences. Shweder and Bourne (1982) describe the tendency in the Eastern cultures of not separating or distinguishing the individual from the social context as a 'sociocentric' conception of relationships,

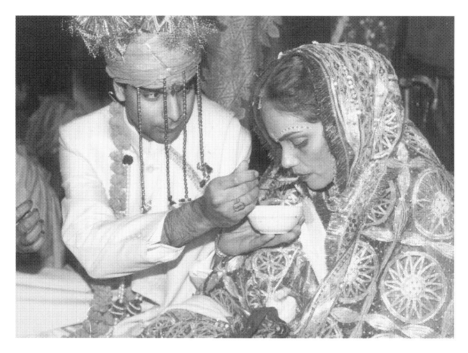

Figure 6.1: Feeding each other, as an important aspect of the wedding ritual.

in contrast to the 'egocentric' conception in the Western cultures. 'In Western cultures, individuality is the prime value and relatedness is secondary . . .' (Tamura and Lau 1992, p 30). Child-rearing practices are the most important manifestations of such cultural ideologies.

To make sense of the child-rearing practices in the Indian culture, it is useful to look at its ideological history. In India, between the 8th and the 5th century BC, a number of heterodox schools emerged to challenge the well-established authority of the Vedas (Table 6.1). Of these, Buddhism had the greatest impact and it spread not only in India but far and wide abroad. It revealed the illusory nature of self or ego and developed practical (meditative and psychosocial) ways of realising freedom from self (Dwivedi 1992, 1994a,b). Such an ideal became an integral part of the Eastern cultures and even the later revival of Hinduism in India contained this ideal within it. Thus, the development of social structures in India was greatly influenced by such an ideology (Dwivedi 1993a, 1994c).

Independence versus dependability

Independence is one of the most cherished ideals in the Western cultures and it permeates all aspects of life, including parenting and psychotherapy. Parents are usually at pains to make their children independent as quickly as possible. This is reflected not only in sleeping arrangements for their babies but also in the encouragement of their children to have and express their own opinions, views and voices. The Eastern cultures, on the other hand, have placed more emphasis on 'dependability' as their cherished ideal (Roland 1980). Parents are often at pains to ensure their dependability. This is reflected in indulgence, prolonged babyhood, immediate gratification of physical and emotional needs, continuous physical closeness and common sleeping arrangements. The idea is to create an atmosphere whereby children can model on their parents and cultivate dependability. The process is seen to be successful when they grow up to become model, dependable 'parents' not only for their children but also for their elderly parents. For an elderly person in the Western culture, the idea of living with their grown-up children is usually associated with the feeling of being a burden on them and can become a source of intense shame and guilt. In the Eastern cultures, it is a source of great joy and pride that one has nurtured one's children in such a way that they have now become truly dependable (Vatuk 1990; Dwivedi 1996a,b,c).

Place of extended family in transcending narcissism

Another aspect of the social structure which helps in overcoming or transcending self or narcissism is the effort to make the institution of extended family a success. The tendency of love is to flow towards one's own and, therefore, extended families can easily break around nuclear family boundaries unless an extra effort is made so that love begins to flow across such nuclear family boundaries (Kakar 1981). A mother in such a family would give affection and food to other children before her own and the children are encouraged to share food and play materials. When they go out they carry each other's children and in conversation 'your' child would mean 'their' child and 'their' child would mean 'yours' (Trawick 1990).

Food and the influence of the Ayurvedic system of medicine

Food is not just food, it also has medicinal qualities. The medicinal values of a number of traditional Indian foods and herbs are now being studied with very encouraging results (Dwivedi S 1996). Most Indian foods and herbs have already been examined by Ayurveda. Ayurveda (literally translated as the science of life) has been a popular medical system in India since the 8th century BC. It is described as a holistic system. It aims to manage life in such a way as to prevent disease and prolong life. This was an oral tradition, which was then documented from the 1st century AD, and there are extensive texts available for each of its eight branches. The rise of Buddhism in India also corresponded with the golden period of Ayurveda (Clifford 1984).

At the heart of Ayurvedic thinking is the concept of a humoral system, i.e. a network of interconnections between food, time, geography, drugs, seasons, temperament and behaviours. Later arrival of the Unani (Greek) system of medicine along with Islam in the Indian subcontinent brought a similar humoral conception. Thus, the Ayurvedic and Unani system of medicine in India must have had an enormous impact on her food habits. Observance of certain rules regarding food, such as Parhej derived from Ayurvedic medicine, has traditionally been an essential code of practice. These are supposed to be observed in order to maintain good health and to get rid of specific illness (Rai and Dwivedi 1988). Thus feeding someone, and in particular a pregnant or lactating mother and her child, needs a great deal of care involving a range of traditional cultural and family specific customs and also the availability of certain foods and their properties.

Social dislocation, racism and food

Most ethnic minority families in the UK have experienced social dislocation some time during their current or previous generations. This has meant not only being exposed to unfamiliar ways of doing things but also a loss of extended family, other important social networks and institutions, such as schools, neighbourhood, distant relatives, film and other media. All of these things offered support and comfort in times of need and reinforced their cultural values. Many have experienced this dislocation as extremely traumatic, especially those who have been expelled from their countries as a result of political turbulence. Experiences of racism, both in the form of racial disadvantages and physical and verbal aggression, have also been the norm for many, along with the feeling that their cultures and value systems are undermined by the major institutions, even poisoning their children's minds. Goldberg and Hodes (1992) highlight how self-poisoning by many Asian adolescent girls symbolises the acting out of the dominant culture of the ethnic majority group that the minority is 'poisonous' or 'harmful'.

Most toddlers in ethnic minority families develop a taste for and relish the food usually prepared in their families, but as they begin to attend school, they take on their peer group's (and sometimes their school staff's) negative attitudes towards ethnic minority foods. Similarly, children from vegetarian families often begin to insist on becoming non-vegetarian. Many parents give in to their children's wishes but find it difficult to make the same emotional investment in these food dishes or to make these foods overflow with their love. In some families, conflicts around food can create difficulties. These sorts of conflicts (which are, of course, both internal and external) often give rise to the types of feeding problems encountered by healthcare professionals.

The role of professionals

In the Western culture, as has already been discussed, there is an emphasis on individuality as the prime value, rather than relatedness. Often teachers, social workers, counsellors and various health professionals, because of their cultural conditioning, tend to perceive their role as that of facilitating individuality, self-expression and independence. An adolescent or a child not expressing such independent views, likes and dislikes may arouse concern in such a professional and at times, a passionate wish to 'rescue' the youngster with the assumption that their family might be repressive and over-restrictive.

Professional attitudes can have an extensive impact on cultural practices and family relationships in transcultural situations (Dwivedi 1996d,e). This can be illustrated by the attitudinal balance model proposed by Heider (1946, 1958). According to Heider's model, a triadic relationship can be in a state of balance if (a) all the dyads are positive, (b) all the dyads are negative (although a vacuous balance) or (c) one dyad is positive and two dyads are negative. Thus, a triadic relationship is in a state of imbalance if one dyad is negative and the other two are positive. In such a situation, in order to balance the system, either the negative relation should turn into positive or one of the positive relationships has to turn into negative.

For example, the professional and parent may have different attitudes towards certain feeding practices. In such a triadic situation (i.e. professional, parent and feeding practice), if any of the three relationships (such as the relationship between the professional and the cultural practice) is negative, a state of imbalance will be created (Figure 6.2). Things will have to change in

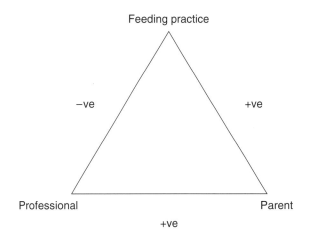

Figure 6.2: A state of imbalance.

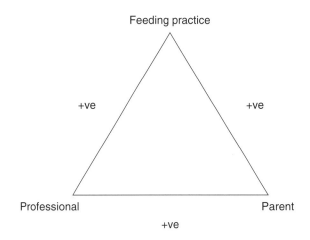

Figure 6.3: A state of balance.

order that a balance can be achieved. There are at least three possibilities: (a) the professional changes their attitude towards the feeding practice (Figure 6.3); (b) the parent changes their attitude towards the feeding practice (Figure 6.4); or (c) the relationship between the professional and the parent changes (Figure 6.5). Similarly, if the relationship between the parent and the professional is negative, it can negatively affect the relationship between child and parent or the child and professional.

The professionals have an important role to play in enhancing parenting skills including those of ethnic minority parents (Dwivedi 1997; Stewart-Brown 1998). Understanding of their cultural context and eliciting of their enthusiasm are, therefore, essential for achieving this (Kemps 1997).

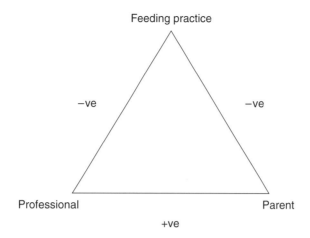

Figure 6.4: Another state of balance.

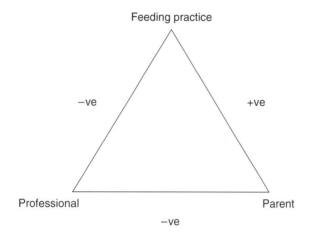

Figure 6.5: Yet another state of balance.

Summary

Food is not just food. In the Indian culture, emotions are grounded in food (as well as in other things) and the attitude towards food and feeding is influenced by the well-established ideologies around the theory of 'Rasa' and 'karma' and of non-self-cherishing. The medicinal values of traditional Indian foods have also been explored by the ancient Indian medical system (Ayurveda). These are again being studied with the help of modern science with very encouraging results (Dwivedi S 1996). Now the Western multinationals have started capitalising on biodiversity, even rushing to patent certain herbal properties that have been traditionally used in the developing and tropical countries.

Many ethnic minority families in the West have also experienced traumatic social dislocation with loss of adequate social, cultural and extended family support, which inevitably impacts on their feeding patterns. Similarly, racism and professional attitudes towards various aspects of their lives, including food, are also bound to influence their feeding and eating practices. In helping ethnic minority families with their children's feeding problems, it is essential for the professionals not only to be aware of but also to be sensitive to the cultural aspects which provide a complex framework in which feeding may be understood.

References

Bennett P (1990) In Nanda Baba's house: the devotional experience in Pushti Marg Temples. In: OM Lynch (ed) *Divine Passions: the social construction of emotion in India*. University of California Press, Berkeley.

Clifford T (1984) *Tibetan Buddhist Medicine and Psychiatry*. Aquarian Press, Wellingborough.

de Bary WT, Hay S, Weiler R and Yarrow A (1958) *Sources of Indian Tradition*. Columbia University Press, New York.

Dwivedi KN (1992) Eastern approaches to mental health. In: T Ahmed, B Naidu and A Webb-Johnson (eds) *Concepts of Mental Health in the Asian Community*, pp 24–30. Confederation of Indian Organisations (UK), London.

Dwivedi KN (1993a) Coping with unhappy children who are from ethnic minorities. In: VP Varma (ed) *Coping With Unhappy Children*, pp 134–51. Cassell, London.

Dwivedi KN (1993b) Emotional development. In: KN Dwivedi (ed) *Group Work with Children and Adolescents: a handbook*. Jessica Kingsley, London.

Dwivedi KN (1994a) The Buddhist perspective in mental health. *Open Mind*. **70**: 20–1.

Dwivedi KN (1994b) Mental cultivation (meditation) in Buddhism. *Psychiatric Bulletin*. **18**: 503–4.

Dwivedi KN (1994c) Social structures that support or undermine families from ethnic minority groups: Eastern value systems. *Context*. **20**: 11–12.

Dwivedi KN (1996a) Culture and personality. In: KN Dwivedi and VP Varma (eds) *Meeting the Needs of Ethnic Minority Children*. Jessica Kingsley, London.

Dwivedi KN (1996b) Children from ethnic minorities. In: V Varma (ed) *Coping with Children in Stress*. Arena Publishers, Aldershot.

Dwivedi KN (1996c) Race and the child's perspective. In: R Davie, G Upton and V

Varma (eds) *The Voice of the Child: a handbook for professionals.* Falmer Press, London.

Dwivedi KN (1996d) Introduction. In: KN Dwivedi and VP Varma (eds) *Meeting the Needs of Ethnic Minority Children.* Jessica Kingsley, London.

Dwivedi KN (1996e) *Meeting the Needs of Ethnic Minority Children.* Transcultural Mental Health On-Line, http://www.priory.com/journals/chneeds.htm

Dwivedi KN (ed) (1997) *Enhancing Parenting Skills.* John Wiley, Chichester.

Dwivedi KN and Gardner D (1997) Theoretical perspectives and clinical approaches. In: KN Dwivedi (ed) *Therapeutic Use of Stories.* Routledge, London.

Dwivedi KN and Prasad KMR (1999) The Hindu, Jain and Buddhist communities; beliefs and practices. In: A Lau (ed) *Asian Children and Adolescents in Britain.* Whurr, London.

Dwivedi R (1996) Community and youth work with Asian women and girls. In: KN Dwivedi and VP Varma (eds) *Meeting the Needs of Ethnic Minority Children.* Jessica Kingsley, London.

Dwivedi S (1996) Putative use of Indian cardio-vascular friendly plants in preventive cardiology. *Annual National Medical Academy of Medical Sciences (India).* **32** (3&4): 159–75.

Geertz C (1973) *The Interpretation of Cultures.* Basic Books, New York.

Goldberg D and Hodes M (1992) The poison of racism and the self poisoning of adolescents. *Journal of Family Therapy.* **14**: 51–67.

Heider F (1946) Attitudes and cognitive organisation. *Journal of Psychology.* **21**: 107–12.

Heider F (1958) *The Psychology of Interpersonal Relations.* John Wiley, New York.

Kakar S (1981) *The Inner World: a psychoanalytic study of childhood and society in India* (2e). Oxford University Press, Delhi.

Kemps CR (1997) Approaches to working with ethnicity and cultural differences. In: KN Dwivedi (ed) *Enhancing Parenting Skills.* John Wiley, Chichester.

Laungani P (1992) Cultural variations in the understanding and treatment of psychiatric disorders: India and England. *Counselling Psychology Quarterly.* **5**(3): 231–44.

Lynch OM (1990a) The social construction of emotion in India. In: OM Lynch (ed) *Divine Passions: the social construction of emotion in India.* University of California Press, Berkeley.

Lynch OM (1990b) The Mastram: emotion and person among Mathura's Chaubes. In: OM Lynch (ed) *Divine Passions: the social construction of emotion in India.* University of California Press, Berkeley.

Marglin FA (1990) Refining the body: transformative emotion in ritual dance. In: OM Lynch (ed) *Divine Passions: the social construction of emotion in India.* University of California Press, Berkeley.

Rai PH and Dwivedi KN (1988). The value of 'Parhej' and 'sick role' in Indian culture. *Journal of the Institute of Health Education.* **16**(2): 56–61

Reat RR (1990) *Origins of Indian Psychology*. Asian Humanities Press, Berkeley.

Roland A (1980) Psychoanalytic perspectives on personality development in India. *International Review of Psychoanalysis.* 1: 73–87.

Shweder RA and Bourne EJ (1982) Does the concept of the person vary cross-culturally? In: AJ Marsella and GM White (eds) *Cultural Conceptions of Mental Health and Therapy.* D Reidel Publishing Company, Dordrecht.

Stewart-Brown S (1998) Evidence based child mental health promotion: the role of parenting programmes. In: KN Dwivedi (ed) *Evidence Based Child Mental Health Care.* Child and Adolescent Mental Health Service, Northampton.

Stocking GW (ed) (1986) *Malinowski, Rivers, Benedict and Others: essays on culture and personality.* The University of Wisconsin Press, Wisconsin.

Tamura T and Lau A (1992) Connectedness versus separations: applicability of family therapy to Japanese families. *Family Process.* **31**(4): 319–40.

Trawick M (1990) The ideology of love in a Tamil family. In: OM Lynch (ed) *Divine Passions: the social construction of emotion in India.* University of California Press, Berkeley.

Vatuk S (1990) To be a burden on others. In: OM Lynch (ed) *Divine Passions: the social construction of emotion in India.* University of California Press, Berkeley.

CHAPTER 7

Family and wider system perspectives

Angela Southall

Introduction: why work with the family?

From the day we are born we are interacting with our environment. Everything we do is part of an interactive process. As children, we develop through this process of interaction, with new knowledge being continually assimilated. The result is a process of constant transformation within and between individuals and relationships. Behaviour, then, does not exist in a vacuum: for every action there is a reaction, with constant feedback between the two, as we adapt to others' responses to us. In other words, this process of being, of interacting, of relating, is a *dynamic* one. Since the context of a young child's behaviour is usually that of the family, the relationships bounded by it and meanings created by it, the family dimension is inevitably all-important. Whatever the theoretical approach, therefore, when there are difficulties a family focus is essential, both in terms of understanding the wider picture and in initiating and sustaining change.

The importance of the family as the 'unit' of treatment is not a new idea, nor even a recent idea. We were being advised by Bowlby as early as 1949 that we should be 'concerned not with children but with the total family structure' when looking at children's problems:

> . . . the overt problem which is brought to the clinic in the person of the child is not the real problem; the problem which as a rule we need to solve is the tension between all the different members of the family.

What Bowlby recognised is that the difficulties experienced by the child cannot be taken in isolation. This is a view that has continued to grow and evolve, with one of its 'shoots' being, of course, the formal discipline of family therapy. Alongside this, there has been an ever-increasing focus on the family at the social and political levels, reflected in recent legislation and policy emphases on parental partnership (e.g. The Children Act 1989). Such an emphasis brings family context to the forefront of considerations for those of us working with children and families, making family-based approaches all the more appropiate.

Of course, there are many different ways of working with families and many different professionals who choose to do family-orientated work. Many of these work in the broad spectrum of health and social care professions and make a distinction between what they do as 'family work' and the formal discipline of family therapy.

This chapter will begin by briefly outlining some of the salient theoretical and methodological perspectives which identify family therapy as a distinct approach. It will then go on to discuss how these ideas are incorporated into practical work with families where there are feeding difficulties. The wider-system perspective is also considered as especially important where there is multiprofessional involvement, as is commonly the case with complex feeding problems.

Although this chapter will be written from a 'formal' family therapy perspective, it has the broad aim of being informative and helpful to anyone wishing to take more of a family focus in their own work, as well as challenging to those who don't! Its aim will be to give a 'flavour' of family therapy, providing something of a framework in which to think about feeding and feeding-related issues, as well as some illustrations of applications of this way of working to feeding problems.

Family therapy as a distinct approach

Defining family therapy is a daunting task. To describe it in a way that approaches completeness would require several chapters or perhaps an entire book in itself. In the limited space available, the aim is to try to convey the essence of this way of working by selecting out key concepts and techniques and by giving examples of the work, rather than focusing on 'what is family therapy'.

Basically, family therapy has as its fundamental concern the person as a whole. Central to this whole-person view is the concept of the 'system', which is defined by the connectedness of those within it and by enduring patterns of relationships, behaviours and beliefs. Imber-Black (1988) gives the following description:

> Family therapy originated with the idea that an individual's problems
> begin to make a different kind of sense when examined in the context
> of the nuclear and extended family. That idea can be extended into an

even more complex meaningful system, composed of individuals, families and larger systems, existing in a wider social context that shapes and guides mutual expectations, specific interactions and outcomes.

Owing to the focus on systems, family therapy is also known as systemic or systems therapy. Many practitioners prefer to use this term as it is less likely to imply work *only* with families. Family and systemic therapists are, in fact, well known for their work within and between all sorts of systems – schools, hospitals, residential establishments or other professional networks – not just that of the family. Much systemic work is, in fact, to do with problems in professional systems. As Reimers and Street (1993) point out, the systems model is 'a model for analysing and solving problems with any system including but not restricted to the family'.

Despite some similarities and areas of overlap between family therapy and other forms of therapy, there are important differences. Basically, no other therapeutic approach has the same sort of emphasis on the family and its extended relationships. Whereas other approaches may focus on the individuals, couples or groups, family therapy is unique in taking as its 'client' the family system as a whole and using a range of methodologies to achieve change within that system. With its focus on family relationships, such an approach immediately challenges ideas of 'maladjustment' and individual pathology.

An evolving approach

Family therapy is a relatively new discipline developed around the psychodynamic tradition during the late 1960s and early 1970s. Different models of systemic working were adopted by the various 'schools' and there have been several revisions and adaptations of ideas as the discipline continues to grow and develop.

In recent years, there has been a shift away from explanations of problems as self-perpetuating sequences of behaviour to considerations which frame the problem in terms of shared meanings. Constructivist models emphasise that this includes not just the family, but everyone who is involved in thinking about and 'constructing' the problem, including professionals (e.g. Boscolo *et al.* 1987).

The constructivist model may be seen as having its branches, if not its roots, in cognitive psychology and personal construct psychology (Kelly 1955). Procter (1981, 1985) suggests the idea of the family construct system as a framework for organising the thinking and behaviour of family members. The system of family constructs develops over time between family members, constituting a 'common family reality' (Felixas 1990) and incorporates constructs from families of origin as well as from the (sub)cultural system to which the family belongs. Such ideas suggest a focus on helping to make the meaning explicit and intervening in a way that promotes change at this level. Interestingly, this echoes Kelly's earlier view that the key issues for promoting change are not the (therapeutic) interpretations of the therapist but those of the client (i.e. interpretations in meaning).

For the systemic therapist, relationship patterns exist within a framework of beliefs, made up of an amalgam of traditions, myths, prejudices and expectations. The family belief system is both an outcome and an initiator of behaviour. For example, a family with a long history of involvement with social services agencies may tend to repeat patterns of crisis in which they will ask their social worker to take one of the children into care. There may be a belief that this is the only solution to the crisis. The more the family believes this, the more they will use it as a solution next time there is a crisis, and so the process continues (Street 1994).

Family context and feeding

The discussion thus far implies that feeding one's child not only involves the giving of food, but also encompasses a huge interactive area of emotions, beliefs, behaviours, social and cultural pressures. All of these things impact on family relationships and may make feeding difficult. Since the parents have the primary responsibility for feeding the child, the greatest impact is on their relationship with the child. To focus in a mechanistic way on food or weight only is to deny the importance of the relationship. Unfortunately, this can happen only too readily once the professional system is accessed: too often, there is a focus on food, rather than the feeding, on weight rather than on relationships.

With the birth of their first baby, the mother and father cease to be a couple and become, with their new child, a family. They have to adjust to their new roles and new definitions about themselves, as they create a new story for themselves about their family. Feeding even a new baby involves, either directly or indirectly, other members of the family. Later, this involvement becomes even more direct, with meal times serving an important family function. Meal times have long served as regulators of family life; often they are the only times that all family members are together. They are occasions when family roles and tasks become defined and where not only is food made and shared together but so, too, are conversations and experiences. Meal times therefore serve important functions in practical, social and meaning-making terms.

Working creatively with the family

The preference of the family or systemic therapist is usually to see the family together, at least initially, to get a sense of the relationships. Although every effort would be made to do this, it is not the case that family therapists see all of the family together all of the time. In troubled families, it has been found most helpful, initially, to see whoever decides to come. Where there are feeding difficulties this often means seeing the parents or carer separately to begin with.

In some families, this may mean working with the parents who are struggling with their child's feeding in the child's absence. Perhaps the child is being fostered or is a hospital inpatient, or perhaps it has been agreed that some work needs to be done without the child being present. Some excellent work may be done on their parenting and their experiences of being parented, which are wholly connected to the present difficulties. They may agree to undertake tasks which either directly or indirectly involve the feeding of their child. Contrary to popular opinion, family therapists *do* see individuals and a number of authors have written on this subject (e.g. Boscolo and Bertrando 1996).

Many systemic therapists working with families where there are feeding problems find themselves meeting initially with the mother. The notion of mothers having the responsibility to feed their families is embedded within many cultures, along with that of personal failure when there is a problem. Not only does the mother often identify it as 'her' problem but others do too, explicitly or not, often by framing it in terms of some kind of a failure in the mother–child relationship.

The family interview

Many who choose family or systemic therapy as an approach do so not only because of its effectiveness; they also value respectful ways of working with people and believe that this approach offers such a way by virtue of its openness towards and appreciation of the family's perspective. There is also an emphasis on therapy as not being about 'doing things to' a family but rather as a process of negotiation between the therapist and family (Dallos and Trelfa 1993). For some, this is a prime motivating factor. Great care is taken nowadays to reassure families that an invitation to come to be seen together is given not because the family are seen as 'the problem'; rather, they are being seen as part of the solution, and a very important part at that. This is always a very important message to get across to families at the first meeting, particularly parents who may feel – understandably – sensitive about being 'blamed' for the problem.

Family-focused approaches are usually concerned primarily with the here and now and this is especially true for family therapy. At the initial meeting, the focus will be on what is happening now with regard to eating and meal times in the family and on helping the family to tell their story of what is the problem and what has led to the present situation. Questions are framed to raise everyone's awareness of relationships and sequences of events. There is an emphasis on questioning in family therapy which arises from the recognition that *how* you ask the question is important, not just what you ask. Although there will undoubtedly be some discussion of past events and some sharing of family stories, for the most part there will be a 'past-into-present' focus in terms of how past experiences have helped to shape present roles and behaviours. For example, there may be some useful exploration of how childhood experiences of being parented have contributed to cognitive constructs around parenting as well as parenting practices themselves. The following exerpt is from a conversation with the parents of Lauren, a very selective eater:

> Mother: 'In our house, we always had to eat everything on the plate. It was almost a sin to leave food to go to waste. My mother had a saying, 'waste not, want not'. I think that, looking back on it, she saw it as her responsibility to get everyone to eat up all their food. I can see that I've taken on this job for myself! I always swore that I would do things differently but I can see that, actually, I'm doing the same thing.'

This conversation continued as follows, with the therapist wondering aloud what might be some of the reasons for doing the same thing.

> Mother: I don't know. It's just what a mother does.
> Therapist: All mothers do this?
> Mother: Well, good mothers (laughs).

The therapist was then able to reflect that a good mother is one who gets her child to eat.

> Therapist: (to father) What effect do you think having that belief might have on Sue when it comes to Lauren's feeding?
> Father: (long pause) I think she probably feels like a complete failure. I think we both do, really, but it's got to affect Sue more than me, because she's the mother . . .

Here, careful questioning helped elicit a powerful belief in *both* parents that a good mother is one who can get her child to eat (and a child has to be 'got' to eat). By definition, therefore, a mother who 'can't' do this has to be bad. The parents felt that this belief was held by the extended family, particularly both grandmothers by whom the mother felt constantly undermined. The more undermined and disempowered she felt, the more effort she put into 'trying to get it right'. This, in turn, affected the way she approached Lauren, leading Lauren to experience meal times as even more aversive. Predictably, she responded by eating less.

In families such as Lauren's, there is usually a strong sense of hopelessness by the time they come into contact with one of the specialist helping agencies. The tendency to feel hopeless and helpless in the face of an enduring problem has been well documented in the mental health literature. As a result, a number of therapeutic approaches have emphasised the importance of helping people to challenge their thinking as a key to helping to change behaviour. One of the ways of doing this is to avoid the common trap awaiting helpers, namely that of focusing too much on what has gone wrong and not enough on what has gone right. This approach serves to exacerbate feelings of helplessness and inadequacy. The alternative is to side-step the problem-focus trap and to have instead the sort of conversation that is more orientated towards solutions. In Lauren's case, this meant that the questioning looked for 'unique outcomes' that contradicted the 'bad mother' story, which was so dominant for them.

Questions that are solution focused rather than problem focused and those that pinpoint unique outcomes tend to be most effective in helping to challenge dominant stories such as this one. This mother, for example, failed to give herself credit for having managed her younger daughter's feeding very well, so that there was neither conflict nor concern about her eating. However, through a process of considered questioning, both parents agreed that their experiences with Lauren had, indeed, made them 'more expert' at feeding their second daughter. The father agreed that the mother had become even more expert than him.

In addition to 'engaging', validating, information gathering and exploring, assessment also involves determining which other, outside, systems are involved and what relationship family members have with them. This is essential in determining who might come to meetings and can form the first stage of an intervention at the professional system level, an illustration of which is given later in this chapter.

Awareness of difference: looking through different lenses

A number of writers and practitioners have emphasised the influence of cultural factors on families and on helpers (*see* Chapters 6 and 14). Baker (1999) writes of the importance of being able to adopt a 'cultural lens' when working with families of a different culture.

This point is well illustrated by my own memory of meeting with the parents of an 11-year-old Asian girl with long-standing feeding problems. Sadia had been admitted to hospital aged five for food refusal and despite the enduring focus on her eating there had been very little change. At age 11 she was a highly selective eater with an extremely small appetite, a tiny child who, nevertheless, managed to eat just enough to remain in reasonable health.

The parents were very involved with their daughter's eating and such was their anxiety to get it right that they had also begun spoon-feeding their eight-year-old son (who was, in fact, very well grown). On spending some time in conversation with them, it emerged that with each successive episode of professional help, Sadia's eating seemed to get worse. This ensured that the parents not only continued to focus on it but they became more and more anxious and had resorted to coercion, force feeding and other aversive methods to try to get their daughter to eat.

As I talked to the parents about what sorts of things had been tried, I became aware of an overwhelming sense of frustration: they did not seem to want to talk about it, only to talk to me about the future. I was puzzled about this and by a sense that we were speaking different languages. I was to discover that we were, of course: as a white woman I had not been able to appreciate their fears for Sadia's future, which were that her slimness would render her unable to have children and she would therefore be rejected by her future husband. Somehow, this story, if heard at all, did not seem to have been thought worthy of further exploration by any of those who had tried to help the family.

The issue of awareness (or lack of it) of difference when meeting families is highlighted by Baker (1999), who describes attempting to retain a systemic awareness by viewing client, family and difficulties through three different 'lenses': one's own professional lens; the lens of differing cultures; and the lens of the larger social system. Sadia's is a good example of what happens without that awareness. It emphasises the need to attend to cultural factors, in order both to be able to hear the family's story and to add to our own understanding as helpers.

Employing an externalising language

Although it is by no means the sole province of family and systemic therapists, they have in recent years emphasised externalisation as a powerful technique for promoting change (e.g. White 1984, 1986, 1988–89; Epston 1986). The basic tenet of such a technique is that the personification or objectification of a problem places it 'out there', rather than inside one particular individual. A famous example is Michael White's use of 'Sneaky Poo' when helping children with soiling problems: the whole family can be enlisted in the fight against

'Sneaky Poo', who is terrorising them all. Identifying a difficulty as outside of a person or family creates an immediate cognitive shift in terms of guilt, blame and 'ownership' of the problem: it not only makes it easier to talk about it, it also makes us think differently about it.

As Parry and Doan (1994) explain:

> Problem externalisation involves talking about *problems* as problems rather than *people* as problems.

Many systemic practitioners would agree with Parry and Doan that it is possible to employ an 'externalising language' from the very start of therapeutic contact. For example, there is an important difference in asking the question 'Can you tell me when Lauren started to have feeding problems?' and an externalising question, such as 'How long do you think you have all been struggling with this feeding problem?'. Externalising conversations often personify the 'problem', as in White's example, above. One example might be talking with a family about the feeding monster who keeps muscling in on family life, no matter what they do to try to keep him out. This way of talking and thinking about difficulties, although on the face of it quite simple and straightforward, contrasts with the traditional way of thinking about people's problems. Parry and Doan (1994) summarise this as follows:

> Although this seems quite a simple notion, it is in direct contrast to the dominant 'mental health story', which pathologises people via placing their problems inside of them.

Adam: a systemic approach to selective eating

Adam was referred to us at three years for help with very selective eating, where he would eat only a certain brand of chocolate bar, bread and butter, and plain crackers and would drink only lemonade. He was in poor health, with frequent 'minor' ailments, coughs, colds and tummy upsets. He was also anaemic and receiving an iron supplement in syrup form, with which he was 'force fed'. Although a small, slight child, Adam's weight remained fairly stable and was not a cause for concern.

In common with many families, it was the mother who attended the first appointment, even though the invitation had been explicit in including both parents or carers and whoever lived at home. The father's involvement was elicited by persevering in inviting him through carefully worded letters. When we met, it was evident that there was parental conflict not only about Adam's feeding but also in terms of the general approach to bringing him up. The father, who was in the forces, took a more traditional 'hard line', whereas the mother took the opposite approach. One of her core beliefs about parenting was that parents should strive not to 'upset' their children. The parents' relationship was complementary in that the more the father toughened up, the more gentle the mother became. It was not known whether this complementarity preceded the feeding difficulties or resulted from them. Certainly, by the time we met they had become very stuck in a cycle in which Adam's poor feeding led them to take an ever stronger position on this 'see-saw'. The pattern was that the mother would seek 'expert' help from a range of healthcare professionals, while the father's view was that these professionals were there as a source of support for the mother, confirming to him that she could not cope. However, he also saw them as not helping. The result was that he distanced himself from them and took up an even 'tougher' position with regard to his son's feeding. It is easy to see how the outside systems therefore contributed to this cycle. The mother was, in fact, quite depressed and isolated, the enforced mobility of the father's work limiting opportunities for maintaining her social and support networks. Helping everyone to shift from their 'stuck' positions therefore involved both the coordination and partnership with professionals in other systems with regard to the feeding difficulties and the separation of the issue of support for the mother (via a community nurse counsellor). Involving the father was an essential first step in trying to effect the movement in the parents from complementarity to a more symmetrical relationship.

Adam's eating progressed slowly, with evening meals being focused upon as a time for the family to come together and eat together. Adam was offered a little of what his parents were eating (something that necessitated a great deal of compromise, as both parents were fairly insistent that their meals were 'unsuitable' for Adam). Previously, meal times had simply not happened. Adam had been fed whenever he had expressed any hunger. He was given food wherever he happened to be, in a very functional way. Neither his father nor mother ate with him, although they did eat together 'sometimes' when Adam was in bed. Having a meal time when the family ate together introduced a structure and routine that they all began to enjoy and that enabled *both* parents to participate in meal-time preparation. It also changed the context of the eating, from being purely functional to being a more relaxed, social time.

It was initially very hard for the parents when there was not an immediate improvement in Adam's eating and when he chose not to sit with them for very long. They were encouraged to persist, however, and acknowledged that the alternative strategy (which they had given a good try) did not work.

Adam's parents were also encouraged to give themselves 'time off' from being parents by getting a babysitter so that they could go out together. This, too, had not been happening. No doubt this was another factor which led to them being able to be more united in their management of Adam generally.

Adam's eating improved and he became more adventurous in trying new foods. He continues to be clear about his likes and dislikes, however, and remains what many parents would call a 'fussy' eater. Adam's parents admit that they would still like him to eat more but their lives are not dominated by his eating in the way that they once were. They have other things to do and think about. They are now expecting another baby.

The family–professional system

Some of the most important work done by family therapists has been by way of informing us that it is not possible to stand outside the family system as an independent observer. Professionals working with families become part of what is known as the family–professional system. Professionals bring with them their own stories about feeding, based on their own life experiences. These will invariably have an impact on the situation with which they are helping, just as the situation will help reshape their stories. Furthermore, the processes taking place in the family–professional system echo those in the family, with similar types of coalitions being established. A common observation is that the professional system can 'mirror' the family one. For example, one might find a family with a different helper forming a coalition with either parent, taking a complementary position to each other and becoming ever more anxious and hostile towards each other. The very emotive nature of feeding problems inevitably adds considerably to the tension and complexity in the situation.

Families with feeding difficulties and multiple helpers

Many families with feeding difficulties have a great many helpers. Children with medical problems, who are premature or who have feeding problems from birth can be said to be born into a system of multiple helpers. It is not unusual for there to be several healthcare professionals, such as a paediatrician, community paediatric nurse, health visitor and dietician, as well as a social worker (sometimes more than one), speech therapist and clinical psychologist. At other times play therapists, child psychotherapists or child psychiatrists may also be involved. Often, the anxiety of the parents is mirrored in the professional system in such a way as to lead them to invite more and more professionals to join them. Furthermore, professional culture expectations support this. As Imber-Coppersmith (1985) notes:

> Our present culture supports the entry of multiple helpers, first by promoting specialisation which identifies a specific kind of helper for

every aspect of a problem . . . and second by deeming that helpers do their job well when they uncover a multiplicity of problems to address.

Multiple helpers may be engaged routinely by families over time, sometimes over generations, as 'their way' of responding to crises. The helpers may fulfil a variety of roles for the family.

However, the situation often gets worse as more helpers are involved: the greater the number of professional helpers, the more helpless the family feels. Among professionals, there may be competing and conflicting beliefs, allegiances, affiliations and proffered solutions.

One of the strengths of the family or systemic therapist is in helping to acknowledge and explore some of these conflicts in a way that is professionally non-threatening. This is achieved by focusing on processes rather than problems, an openness to adopt a number of positions and alternative viewpoints, and by using techniques such as externalisation, already described, which separates the problem from the individual helper and places it 'outside', where it becomes something for everyone to work on. This type of contribution of family therapy to working more effectively with larger systems is described by Imber-Coppersmith (1985):

> Applying the systemic model to families and multiple helpers has widened the conceptual base for understanding human problems. Just as family therapy initially provided a move away from individual blame concepts, so the family–multiple helpers view provides a move away from family blame concepts. The attempt here is not to blame professionals but rather to grasp the complexities that evolve when families and multiple helpers interact . . .

Such an approach encourages a mutual curiosity about one another's place in the macrosystem, enabling movement from hostile or negative views of other helpers. It also emphasises the therapist as part of the system, rather than outside it. Many find that the work in the professional system is not only an important prerequisite to working with the family but essential in helping what may be a 'stuck' situation. Only then can things begin to move forward.

Example of a professional system intervention with a tube-fed child

Matthew was referred at three years. He was in long-term foster care and had been tube-fed since his reception into local authority care two years previously on 'failure to thrive' grounds. He was the subject of a child protection order and was on the child protection register on the grounds of physical abuse and neglect. There had been several previous attempts by other agencies to help with Matthew's feeding with no success. Typically, those who had become involved had stayed involved, resulting in a huge professional system. Different agendas, emphases and working practices made the ground ripe for conflict. The professional groupings were characterised by poor communication and conflict, with open hostility between some professional groups, each blaming the other for the failure to make any progress.

Each successive failure meant that the foster parents became increasingly regarded with suspicion. There had even been suggestions from medical professionals that Matthew's case was an example of Munchausen's syndrome by proxy. This created conflict between the social services and medical systems. The foster parents, for their part, found themselves in a complementary relationship with the outside systems: the more help they were offered, the more helpless and defeated they became. Their increasing anxiety and confusion made them less inclined to cooperate, thus creating further suspicion and frustration in the medical system.

The author became involved following a referral from the hospital paediatrician. Although there was an army of helpers already attached to Matthew and his carers, there was not, at that point, any involvement of the service to which I belonged. The referral was probably an attempt to redress this 'oversight' and lack of inclusiveness by involving yet another professional.

The programme

To change the parents' position vis-à-vis the 'expert' systems

The first part of the intervention consisted of a meeting with the foster parents on their own. This was, in itself, difficult to arrange and necessitated careful and sensitive negotiation with other professionals, some of whom insisted that they needed to come, too. At the initial meeting, great care was taken to listen to the parents and value what they said. It was explained that this meeting was to agree on a strategy to help Matthew. It was then suggested that as there were so many people involved it was necessary to have a 'core' group representing the 'feeding experts': this would be the parents, therapist and dietician. Although we would all be meeting together to discuss Matthew's progress, no one else would call at the house and no one else would give advice. The parents' response to this was a mixture of surprise, relief and apprehension. Although they clearly felt swamped by all of the help they were receiving and expressed a keenness to see fewer people and have fewer appointments, they had also got used to having a lot of helpers.

The meeting of the family–professional system

This was followed by a meeting of the family and professional system, during which the rationale for having the core group was explained and the flow of information and coordination of different services were negotiated. This meeting proved to be the most fundamental component of the plan to help Matthew and his family. An important function of this meeting was to help the professionals to hold their own feelings of anxiety and impatience for change.

Physically, having a large group of professionals in the room together can be a powerful way of making a statement. The response from the professionals is invariably 'I never realised there were this many of us'. As a facilitator, it is often useful to make the point to the family: 'I can't believe there are this many people involved with Matthew's feeding. How ever do you manage to talk to us all?'

The externalising language, mentioned earlier, which is so helpful to families and individuals is also extremely useful when working with larger systems. A conversation employing this way of thinking and talking about the problem enabled those present to move from defensiveness about what was perceived as their own therapeutic failures. This was a focus from the onset, with helpers asked to introduce themselves in terms of their relationships with Matthew and his family and then to say something about the way they had been helping with the feeding problem. The effectiveness of this technique has already been highlighted. It is important to note that this is also the case for groups, where it can have similarly powerful effects, as summarised below (from White 1988–89):

- it decreases conflict between people over who is responsible for the problem
- it reduces the sense of failure people have in not having solved the problem
- it unites people against the problem, rather than against each other
- it frees people to think about the problem in different ways.

To have a 'core group' meeting to plan/clarify the feeding regime

By carefully limiting professional involvement there was automatically less advice giving. At the same time there was acknowledgement of the foster parents' coping and the skills they had developed during the period they had been caring for Matthew. Through a process of consulting with them as experts on Matthew's feeding, the meetings became a process of empowering them, as well as offering support and encouragement on a practical level.

A key moment in therapy came when the foster mother informed us with great pride of a change she had made: previously, she would not have felt confident enough to initiate this change without consulting the health professionals 'in charge'; she now felt expert enough in her own right. The core group continued to follow the agreed plan together, using a combined approach based loosely on behavioural management techniques and 'shaping up' Matthew's feeding while maintaining an overarching systemic focus. This enabled Matthew to gradually resume oral feeding. The process was long, taking about 10 months in all.

As can be seen from the above description, the plan for helping Matthew (as well as Adam and Lauren) involved attending to both meaning and behavioural change. Dallos and Trelfa (1993) remind us that people engage in thinking and behaving simultaneously and caution against giving one primacy over the other. Furthermore, there is, of course, a reciprocal relationship between the two, with beliefs influencing our behaviour and behaviour, in turn, affecting our thoughts, attitudes and beliefs. For this reason, they suggest that therapy must inevitably involve both:

> A helpful re-frame should lead to behavioural change which can lead to further conceptual change. Likewise, a behavioural task, such as the parents changing roles for a week, should also lead to new ways of seeing events, new behaviours . . . new constructions and so on.

Story revision: how would you like things to be?

Recent systemically orientated practice has been very much influenced by a school of therapy arising out of the constructivist domain, known as narrative therapy. One of the important and challenging emphases of the narrative therapists is on what they term 'story revision'. Although there continue to be parallels with cognitive psychology, the introduction of the narrative dimension brings to bear a richness and many-layered influence. Parry and Doan (1994) have this to say:

> The introduction of the narrative dimension . . . has taken the theme of the limits of perspective a step further. It emphasises that whether the viewer is a person, a family, a community or a people, the world is unavoidably viewed through a succession of stories – not only a personal story, but gender, community, class and cultural stories.

The narrative therapists point out the importance of 're-storying' as an essential part of the helping process. Parry and Doan (1994) suggest that those of us in the so-called 'helping professions' need to be aware of the limits and pitfalls of our training. They suggest that we are very good at analysing things and taking them apart, but less good at putting them back together:

> We have been increasingly concerned that, to a large extent, our training has inadvertently predisposed us . . . to be much better at story deconstruction than at story revision. This is especially true of training that attempts to emulate the medical science model.

Parry and Doan make a strong case for the importance of story revision, warning against leaving those 'deconstructed' clients in a state of 'psychological freefall' (i.e. the problem has been well and truly taken apart but scant attention has been paid to life without it). For those of us involved with helping families resolve their feeding problems, this means that the end point is not the resolution of the feeding problem but the reconstruction of the episode.

In practical terms, this entails enabling the family to construct a new story about themselves and about the problem, perhaps as an ongoing process throughout. For example, Lauren's parents were able to move from a position of seeing themselves as parental failures with a 'sick' child to that of having become expert at feeding their children and having a very independent daughter with strong views of what she liked and disliked. Matthew's foster parents moved from a similar story of being inadequate to one of being expert enough to 'sort out' the experts. Interestingly, when they retell their story, they now recall that they were 'chosen' to parent Matthew because of their skill in managing tube-fed children (which was the case, but somewhere along the line this became forgotten).

The emphasis in family therapy methodology on how questions are asked remains. There are questions which help re-story the past and have the effect of immediately facilitating a different way of thinking about past events and one's part in them. For example, 'Despite having a really difficult few years, you have managed to find ways of helping Lauren to become much more confident about making choices. What do you think other people would say about you that made it possible for you to get to this point?' It is important to remember, as Epston (1993) emphasised, that 'each time we ask a question, we are generating a possible version of life'.

Summary

This chapter has emphasised the importance of working with the family and has outlined some of the useful ways that family or systemic therapies can be applied to helping families with feeding problems. It highlights the importance of being able to take account of and be responsive to other professional systems and demonstrates that interventions at this level can often be very powerful and effective. It introduces the important dimension of 'us' as professionals and means that we have to consider our part in the drama. It also raises the issue of helping people to reconstruct their stories, often the very point at which many helpers exit the stage. Overall, the chapter has, hopefully, reflected some of the richness and diversity of systemic working as well as the complexity of issues related to feeding. The whole picture is not only rarely seen but is rarely even looked for. This may be an unfortunate by-product of our 'expertness', against which we must remain eternally vigilant:

> There is a strong, historically dominant story in our culture that true understanding involves being able to reduce something to its essential elements. This can be a very useful model for many areas of interest, but in dealing with the problems that humans encounter in the process of living, a wide angle lens is often more useful (Parry and Doan 1994).

References

Baker KA (1999) The importance of cultural sensitivity and therapist self-awareness when working with mandatory clients. *Family Process.* **38**(1): 55-67.

Boscolo L and Bertrando P (1996) *Systemic Therapy with Individuals.* Karnac Books, London.

Boscolo L, Cecchin G, Hoffman L and Penn P (1987) *Milan Systemic Family Therapy: conversations in theory and practice.* Basic Books, New York.

Bowlby J (1949) The study and reduction of group tensions in the family. *Human Relations.* **II**(2).

Dallos R and Trelfa J (1993) To be or not to be: family beliefs, madness and the construction of choice. *Journal of Family Therapy.* **4**(3): 63–82.

Epston D (1986) Night watching: an approach to night fears. *Dulwich Centre Review.* 28–39.

Epston D (1993) Internalising discourses versus externalising discourses. In: S Gilligan and R Price (eds) *Therapeutic Conversations.* Norton, New York.

Felixas G (1990) Approaching the individual, approaching the system: a constructivist model for integrative psychotherapy. *Journal of Family Psychology.* **4**(1): 4–35.

Imber-Black E (1988) *Families and Larger Systems: a family therapist's guide through the labyrinth.* Guilford Press, New York.

Imber-Coppersmith E (1985) Families and multiple helpers: a systemic perspective. In: D Campbell and R Draper (eds) *Applications of Systemic Therapy.* Grune and Stratton, London.

Kelly GA (1955) *The Psychology of Personal Constructs*, vols 1 and 2. Norton, New York.

Parry A and Doan RE (1994) *Story Revisions: narrative therapy in the post-modern world*. Guilford Press, New York.

Procter H (1981) Family construct psychology: an approach to understanding and treating families. In: S Walrond-Skinner (ed) *Developments in Family Therapy: theories and applications since 1948*. Routledge, London.

Procter H (1985) A personal construct approach to family therapy and systems interventions. In: E Button (ed) *Personal Construct Theory and Mental Health*. Croom Helm, London.

Reimers S and Street E (1993) Using family therapy in child and adolescent services. In: J Carpenter and A Treacher (eds) *Using Family Therapy in the 90s*. Blackwell, Oxford.

Street E (1994) A family systems approach to child-parent separation: 'developmental closure'. *Journal of Family Therapy*. **16**: 347–65.

White M (1984) Pseudo-encopresis: from avalanche to victory, from vicious to virtuous cycles. *Family Systems Medicine*. **2**(2): 150–60.

White M (1986) Negative exploration, restraint and double description: a template for family therapy. *Family Process*. **25**: 169–84.

White M (1988–89) The externalisation of the problem and the re-authoring of lives and relationships. *Dulwich Centre Newsletter*. **Summer**: 3–200.

PART 2

APPLICATIONS

CHAPTER 8

Beginning with breast-feeding: breast-fed infants and their mothers

Mary Smale

Introduction

The initiation of breast-feeding plays a central part in the adjustment of many new parents to their caring role. Currently, 50% of babies in the UK are exclusively breast-fed at discharge, with half of these leaving hospital within 48 hours of birth (Foster *et al.* 1997). The percentage of breast-fed babies is lower than in many other countries, however, and may represent the beginning of a perceived failure for women, as it is often something they intended to do.

This chapter suggests a number of reasons that make it difficult for women to enjoy breast-feeding. Some of these are social and cultural, whereas others relate directly to the medical and healthcare system in which the new mother finds herself. This chapter offers a holistic framework for understanding breast-feeding, considers situations where it may be problematic and examines a range of helping strategies.

Breast-feeding in context

Breast-feeding, accepted as the healthiest means of feeding young babies, is almost invisible in our society. It can be seen as both 'natural' and 'abnormal', and women who choose to breast-feed often experience tensions between expectation and reality. Many 'problems' relate to cultural expectations (e.g. perceptions of mothers 'failing to control their babies' and their own use of time). The speed, rhythm, frequency and duration of breast-feeds are all very important to the other people in the mother's life (e.g. 'non-nutritive' feeding may be condemned as 'using you as a dummy'). Even the phrase 'demand feeding', used for babies' free access to breast milk implies a relationship based on tyranny. These subtle implications may shape the way in which a mother may delay her response to the baby, making feeding more difficult. Although the majority of mothers have nourished their babies successfully in the womb, there is usually conditional expectation of success in doing so after birth. Many mothers feel pressurised to introduce formula milk and/or bottles, and breast-feeding is seen as making mothers vulnerable to physical exhaustion and emotion, neither of which is justified by research.

A situation may arise where physiological responses are interrupted, and at such times mothers are often advised to begin formula-feeding or to supplement breast milk. The example below shows how, by allowing the natural processes to predominate, successful breast-feeding may continue.

A mother heard of a friend's death in a plane crash. As she fed her six-week-old baby she was aware of her distress inhibiting the flow of her milk. She talked to the baby and allowed herself to cry, experiencing little sensation of let-down for two days, but continuing to feed her baby frequently. Her let-down reflex returned to normal and she continued to breast-feed for a year.

Soreness and inadequate milk supply (real or supposed) are given as the main reasons for early discontinuation of breast-feeding by around 25% of these women within the first few weeks (Foster *et al.* 1997). Many of the two thirds of women who begin breast-feeding regret discontinuing. It is claimed that nutritional risk is at its highest at the point of weaning, and this is when feeding problems are most likely to develop (Drewett and Young 1998). It is suggested in this chapter that confidence about later feeding decisions may need to be seen in the context of these challenges.

Isolated breast-feeding clinics (e.g. Oxford's John Radcliffe Hospital) enable women to self-refer for concerns, but most interventions for well babies happen within the context of community midwifery and health visiting services. Concerns relate to the adequacy of breast milk, colic, vomiting and the frequency of breast-feeding. Where pathology is suspected or if the baby is premature, appropriate paediatric staff become involved.

Some health professionals dealing with feeding difficulties in breast-fed babies may have limited training or experience of normal breast-feeding. This is partly because it is a largely invisible activity on paediatric wards, with only one in five of all babies admitted for gastroenteritis being breast-fed (Howie *et al.* 1989). However, understanding how breast-feeding works can be helpful when assessing whether a baby is feeding effectively.

Factors in breast-feeding: research, physiology and culture

Important understandings gained over the last few decades clarify differences between breast-feeding and bottle-feeding (Royal College of Midwives 1991). These are summarised below.

Foremilk and hindmilk

Whereas bottled milk is homogenised, the fat content of breast milk varies diurnally and within each feed from a breast (Hytten 1954). Increasing fat is made available as milk cells are squeezed in response to a surge in hormones causing the let-down reflex. There is not a steep step at let-down between low-fat (fore)milk and high-fat (hind)milk, but a feed-long gradient. Let-down is visible as the baby changes from a short period of quick intermittent sucking to steady deep gulps with normal pausing. It is quite normal for women not to experience it subjectively.

Supply and demand

Research shows that not only is it necessary for milk to be removed for appetite-responsive milk synthesis to continue, but that milk *not* so removed causes the delivery of a message stopping milk production (Renfrew *et al.* 1999). Frequent feeding is normal in breast-fed babies, especially when young, during the evening. Changes in feeding pattern may happen for a few days at a time – the so-called 'growth spurts' – as normal parts of the achievement of balance in demand and milk supply. There is no evidence for the need in normal babies to receive additional liquids. These are known to shorten breast-feeding duration (Renfrew *et al.* 1999).

These understandings are in contradiction to powerful social messages about the need to discipline babies into regular feed times so that babies can be socialised into independence and the mother is as free as possible to resume economically active life. Only 50% of women in the last government survey had attempted to breast-feed publicly (Foster *et al.* 1997). Women can 'solve' such problems by assertiveness, discretion, staying at home or resorting to bottles of expressed breast milk or formula. While some babies cope with a variety of methods of feeding, some find a teat subverts the development of a secure breast-feeding technique. Interventions such as nipple shields and feeds from bottles or cups may have varying effects on different babies and need to be used with the utmost caution (Renfrew *et al.* 1999). Nipple shields reduce milk supply (Woolridge *et al.* 1980). There is current controversy over whether such interventions cause 'confusion', as has been claimed, or whether a baby who has found rewarding attachment difficult is simply choosing to rely on them and not respond to prior instinctive responses. Avoiding bottles until breast-feeding technique is secure in mother and baby seems a wise precaution.

Positioning and attaching the baby in breast-feeding

Recent biomedical orthodoxy emphasises the learning of these skills. It is evident from working with mothers that many babies are not able to get a good enough mouthful of breast tissue to enable milk transfer to be efficient. Tew (1990), arguing against the rationale for the superiority of hospital intervention around the time of birth, questions the assumption that this means all women need remedial education.

> Every other newborn mammal knows instinctively how to find and in its own time make use of its mother's milk-providing nipple and the mother knows instinctively how to facilitate this process . . . these instincts, essential to survival, are assumed to be inactive in the human baby and mother and to need relearning under profes-sional guidance (Tew 1990, p 3).

The work of Righard and Alade (1990) offers one explanation for the puzzle: Westernised birth may be putting most mothers into a 'remedial' category rather than allowing the development of a set of responses in the context of a period of uninterrupted intimacy following birth, as described in Chapter 4.

Babies in normal births

Twenty years ago research found separation of mother and baby for washing and weighing shortened average breast-feeding (de Chateau *et al.* 1977). Observations of mother and baby in skin contact suggest that babies can find the breast and begin breast-feeding after typical behaviours including recovery from the birth, salivating, making characteristic calling sounds, mouthing, rooting and practice feeding on their own hands, within the period of around an hour (Righard and Alade 1990). There is no evidence that this sequence must happen within any arbitrary time limit (Renfrew *et al.* 1999). It is not known how many babies who sleep after a period without such stimulating contact would wish to feed earlier given the opportunity. Such approaches to birth are still not yet common, largely because of cultural barriers such as the perceived need to wash the baby and to communicate birth weight to the family. Pethidine use may mean the baby takes longer to be able to initiate feeding and that mothers will need more help (Rajan 1994). Not only instrumental deliveries but also very quick second stages in delivery may leave babies who find hand or body contact difficult and may choose to sleep rather than feed. A 'hands-off' approach may help here, not only in terms of the helper's avoidance of touching the baby's head, but even offering the breast from above.

Breast milk supply and comfort are compromised by attachment difficulties. The baby does not need to suck on the nipple, causing it trauma, but to strip milk from a teat formed from a considerable amount of breast tissue. This ensures that the nipple is safely held at the back of the baby's mouth so the milk ducts which lie below the areola can be milked by his tongue. The baby actively takes most breast tissue from the part of the breast nearest to his lower lip, at his own pace, enabled by the mother's stimulus of his mouth area and a pushing of his whole body towards hers. Figure 8.1 shows diagrammatic 'stills', which exemplify two ends of a continuum of possible attachment situations. It will not always be easy to tell the 'right' way (a and b) from the less effective (c and d) as mothers' breasts can obscure details. It is more important to observe the dynamic movements implied, rather than to take a 'snapshot' approach and assume all is well. This is especially true when there is pain for the mother, unsettled behaviour in the baby or a slow weight gain.

Figure 8.1a shows a baby with a wide open mouth and, fleetingly glimpsed, a lowered tongue, ready to scoop up a good mouthful of breast tissue for a comfortable and effective feed. The nipple will have been opposite the baby's nose rather than entering the middle of the mouth. This is facilitated by allowing the baby to flex back his or her head so as to approach the breast from below. In Figure 8.1b the lower lip is curled back, the chin is in contact with the breast and the mouth is open at an angle approaching 180 degrees. Figure 8.1c shows a baby approaching the breast with a pursed mouth more appropriate for bottle feeding. In Figure 8.1d a baby is shown taking a limited amount of breast tissue, possibly causing pain to the mother and making it impossible for the baby to strip the milk effectively from inside the breast.

Without the knowledge outlined above it is easy to assume breasts are similar to bottles. For example, mothers who expect the baby to be passive in the process often repeat fast dabbing with the end of the breast, following by the insertion of the nipple. Holding the breast too near the nipple can restrict this active engulfing by the baby. A mother with sore nipples or who cannot cope with the idea of the baby being too close may find this very difficult and hold herself back at the crucial moment as the baby gapes and lunges.

Research is lacking about whether attachment might be best enabled physically or verbally by carers. Reasons for non-invasive interventions include avoiding making mothers dependent on another person's skill in an intrinsically non-medical area of life, and the possibility of distressing the baby by forcing him on to the breast. The Royal College of Midwives recommend a

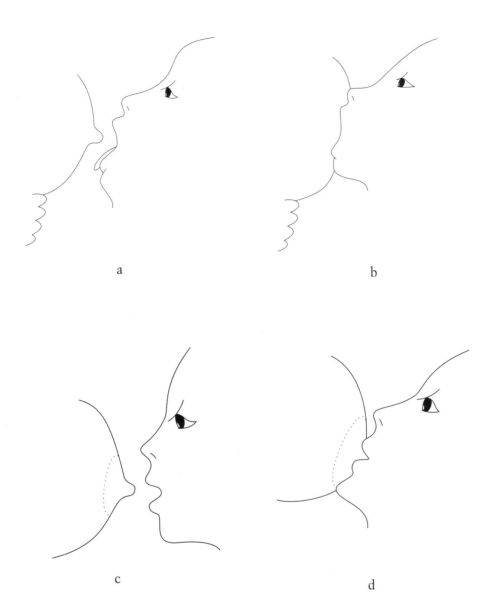

Figure 8.1: Two ends of a continuum of possible attachment situations. (a) and (b) show the right way, while (c) and (d) show the less effective way of attaching the baby to the breast.

verbal approach with physical intervention only if necessary (Royal College of Midwives 1991).

Where there are problems, it is easy to concentrate on the transfer of milk to the baby in a mechanistic way. However, as is clear from the above description, the process is a more subtle one, with more interactions, as is suggested in Chapter 4. Those who experience difficulties several weeks into feeding often describe long delays between birth and an attempt at a first feed, with low initial success and high intervention. However, well-supported and motivated mothers can manage to establish lactation in difficult circumstances such as premature birth. Tube-fed, expressed breast milk may be used for many weeks before breast-feeding is established, which shows that removing time constraints and pressure can be beneficial (Jelliffe and Jelliffe 1978).

Involving the father is important. Currently, it is often the father who is encouraged to 'bond' with the baby in the first hour while the mother receives attention. Many hospitals offer guidelines reinforcing this, suggesting that the more a partner is involved in baby care, the less likely he is to feel 'left out'.

Breast-feeding mothers are encouraged to express their milk so that another person can sometimes give the feed (Manning 1997), although this is only one of the ways in which fathers can become involved in the care of the baby. Informed decision making in this area means that parents need to be told that teats used too early, especially if breast-feeding is not going well, may persuade the baby to opt for the instant 'fix' of a bottle. Parents may find it more helpful for the establishment of breast-feeding for a father to hold and stroke mother and baby together rather than have to accept a part in separating them for any length of time during the period immediately after the birth. The cultural and personal desire to involve a father from the beginning in his baby's life may need to be balanced with the parents' wishes in relation to infant feeding.

Technical details point to an active cooperation between mother and baby in achieving breast-feeding, which sets the tone for later encounters over food. In breast-fed children, timing and appetite control in terms of both quantity and content are decided by the child. When weaned they often show a marked preference for autonomous use of spoons and finger-foods. The following example is a good illustration of a transition from breast-feeding to engaging with other food.

A mother described to me how, after several months of exclusive breast-feeding, she noticed her baby reaching for the pear she was eating. She held it for her and the baby sucked, scraped and gummed her way through nearly all of it with no ill effects. The mother was fascinated by how many skills were in place for this first encounter and that this soft fruit was, of course, sweet and juicy like breast milk.

What mothers bring to the initiation of breast-feeding

'Feeding in mammals in early infancy is social, involving an interaction between the infant and a caretaker, generally the mother' (Drewett and Young 1998). Mothers have a range of expectations in relation to infant feeding, depending on their previous experiences, subjective and vicarious. It can be important to give mothers time to express their feelings in relation to personal and cultural learning.

Little is known of the mother's instinctive response to the feeding behaviour of the normal newborn other than the way in which her nipples become more protractile and her milk is let down for the baby.

What health professionals bring

In the light of cultural sanctions against baby-led breast-feeding and related difficulties in achieving personal 'success' in breast-feeding, it may be difficult for health professionals to enact physiologically based knowledge. Many ideas about breast-feeding have proved resistant to research information. An example is the reluctance to change practice towards continued breast-feeding in the case of diarrhoea, when many doctors advise fasting for babies (Hin-Mang *et al.* 1985). Conflicting advice is not helpful and may distress mothers, for whom a major consideration is to keep professionals happy (Green *et al.* 1988; Smale 1996). Careful use of language helps to avoid transmitting cultural rather than psychological or physiological norms (e.g. one may ask 'Is any pattern beginning to emerge in the baby's needs?' rather than 'Are you getting the baby into a routine?').

The context for initiating feeding

Helpers may have been enabling or uncommunicative, partners supportive or in need of care from the mother. A mother may know – consciously or unconsciously – that she has been nurtured or be unable to feel she is 'full' of anything worth offering to a baby. Each physical or psychological element leaves the mother in a different place in relation to her readiness to respond to her baby's needs and if there are problems, it is worth non-judgementally exploring with her the context in which breast-feeding began. The baby may be the mother's firstborn – amazing the mother with the strength of the first suck. He or she may be a confident or a hesitant 'second chance' feeder. Additionally, the birth can leave the mother physically exhausted, disappointed, euphoric or emotionally drained.

Other factors may also influence the responsiveness of the baby. For example, a stomach full of mucus can beguile a baby into not feeding, while the treatment for jaundice can make babies sleepy. The mother may find such situations frustrating and lose confidence in her ability to satisfy her seemingly unresponsive baby. At the same time, she may also feel that her milk supply is jeopardised or uncomfortably overabundant. It is clear that it is food and not water that metabolises out bilirubin in physiological jaundice, the laxative effect of colostrum and demand feeding being helpful (de Carvalho *et al.* 1981). A need to 'wash out' the baby from the inside may remain in helpers. There is no evidence for deleterious effects on healthy babies from long periods between feeds (Renfrew *et al.* 1999).

Where the mother experiences delays in the initiation of feeding, she and carers may become anxious. There may be an early impetus towards offering formula or seeing breast-feeding as 'treatment' (i.e. a way of getting calories into an unresponsive baby lest he or she become hypoglycaemic or jaundiced). This contrasts with the enjoyment of breast-feeding, as part of a responsive comforting experience for both parties. Medical interventions may also threaten the breast-feeding relationship. A recent paper intended as the basis for a local policy on hypoglycaemia attempts to reduce inappropriate interventions which threaten the breast-feeding relationship (British Association of Perinatal Medicine *et al.* 1997).

Colic, easily confused with the suspicion of an inadequate amount or 'richness' of milk, has been explained in various ways, including dairy product sensitivity and a disproportionate intake of foremilk. This latter theory is well substantiated (Woolridge and Fisher 1988; Evans *et al.* 1995). Birth difficulties are also believed by some to lead to colic. Cranial osteopathy, controversial in the UK, is sometimes used as a treatment, offering parents a route to a greater sense of control over an otherwise distressing situation. Such actions can reassure them that breast-feeding is not in itself causing the problem, as others may suggest.

Psychosocial factors affecting the context of breast-feeding

Mothers who begin breast-feeding have the choice of whether to continue several times each day. Those who persist in breast-feeding despite physical and psychological distress often continue because of the advantages of breast milk. These mothers often speak of their hope that the time (and perhaps the pain) they have 'invested' will bring rewards.

While most women in the UK who find breast-feeding unappealing will currently opt for bottle-feeding, some will find themselves persuaded to attempt breast-feeding on health grounds. They may experience difficulties reconciling their intellectually driven wishes with realities of breast-feeding (e.g. something as basic as the loss of control symbolised by leaking milk between feeds). Barnes *et al.* (1993) suggest that the birth of a child might represent an important loss of control to some mothers. Toleration of the normal pauses in a breast-fed baby's feeding can be low in some mothers who expect unbroken activity.

Body consciousness and self-image

The mother's perception of her body shape has been found to affect the decision to breast-feed (Barnes *et al.* 1993). It is possible that this may also affect the mother's style of breast-feeding as outlined in the example below.

One diet-conscious mother, once technique was improved and her previously very slow-gaining baby showed a slightly above average weight gain, was very concerned lest the infant became obese.

Psychosexual and relationship issues

Deutsch suggested that the possible sensual/sexual feelings associated with breast-feeding were distasteful to women (Deutsch 1945). It is not known to what extent such feelings may interfere with attempted breast-feeding. Even women who have been abused, and where abuse has involved the breasts, may decide to breast-feed on health grounds, although they may find this abhorrent. Issues involving the resumption of intercourse and partners' feelings are well covered in the review by Bam-Yam and Darby (1997). Partners have been identified in research as playing an important role in decision making (White *et al.* 1992; Hewat and Ellis 1986). Partners and significant others may help mothers to persist in breast-feeding (e.g. by encouraging them not to give up in a crisis).

In terms of relationship issues, some of the needs of parents are summarised below. Both parents need:

- good information to understand and experience pain-free and, sometimes, less time-consuming breast-feeding
- to be listened to in a non-judgemental manner, to enable them to make fully informed choices

- encouragement to find time to talk to one another about issues (e.g. ideas about structure, timing of feeding and sleeping, or resumption of a sexual relationship).

Cultural control of time and space in infant feeding

Cultural views regarding time for and control of breast-feeding often extend to insisting that babies achieve three meals a day at a young age. There may be the suggestion to use solids to encourage a diminishing of breast milk intake. Where the baby is slow to accept some or any semi-solid food, mothers may blame themselves or be blamed for breast-feeding too long.

Pathological situations

With premature babies, breast milk (possibly fortified) is regarded as the best choice except in rare cases, because of its anti-infective properties and the mother's early involvement. Breast-milk banks are rare, so pumps, sterilising facilities, the teaching of hand and pump expression and, if required, a private area should be available whether or not the mother remains in hospital.

It is known that breast-feeding mothers value a supportive psychological atmosphere more than bottle-feeding mothers (Wright 1988). Using devices for expressing breast milk so as to monitor production levels of milk is stressful and likely to be misleading. Often the situation of being in an intensive care unit may cause temporary let-down problems, and besides this, babies are usually able to extract more milk than plastic devices. Support from sympathetic staff who believe in the mother's ability to nourish her baby should include reassuring her that any drop in milk supply is due to pump use or low stimulation from the baby, but that the supply will respond as the baby grows.

Other situations linked to feeding problems occur when babies have pressing medical needs, such as those with heart problems, neurological difficulties, Down's syndrome and cleft lip. This often results in parents struggling to establish breast-feeding. Such babies provide extra challenges but also gains from breast-feeding. Rarely, an illness may make breast-feeding impossible (e.g. galactosaemia). Family and friends and sometimes health professionals, while encouraging the offering of breast milk at least initially, may find it difficult to understand why a mother may be so single-minded in her desire to breast-feed once the baby is out of hospital.

Breast-feeding offers comfort to both baby and mother in the recovery from an operation. Both mothers and babies may find the length of time without a feed very distressing during the period prior to and following surgery. However, some authorities suggest that, since breast milk leaves the stomach within one and a half hours, the baby may be fed up to two hours before surgery (Morbacher and Stock 1991). Hence, the time between feeds need not be as great as anticipated. A mother whose baby has been suddenly taken ill may feel a loss of confidence in herself and needs reassurance that her nurturing is valuable and that her milk supply will return after a period of intensive feeding.

Drug treatments rarely prevent breast-feeding, yet there are many drugs where manufacturers are not able to claim full testing. Concerns about the possible hazards of some treatments may become problematic, and the easiest route seems to be to advise the end of lactation. However, the use of alternative drugs may be suggested, and ways of limiting any damage may be found. Support groups usually have access to specialist help in this area.

Any feeding difficulty during breast-feeding affects both members of an intimately linked biologically and psychologically dyadic pair. Even comparatively minor conditions such as a blocked duct – with poor advice to stop feeding – may lead to a mother's weaning.

Not enough milk – social or individual pathology?

Figures from the Office for National Statistics hide a complexity of psychosocial misunderstandings and coercion. Reasons why women end breast-feeding include social ignorance as to the 'normalness' of breast-feeding, which may be carefully encouraged by formula manufacturers (e.g. an emphasis on the need for expensive diet, essential rest and the fragility of breast milk supply). A mother may feel under pressure to bottle-feed if this is seen as a quicker way of getting her baby home from a special care baby unit (Taylor and Littlewood 1994) as is shown in the vignette below.

> A mother returned her breast pump saying the hospital staff had told her that her milk was not growing her baby fast enough for him to be allowed home the next weekend. When she asked what to do with all the milk she knew she would be producing someone suggested she feed it to the cat. Despite being assured that she could maintain lactation and resume breast-feeding when her baby returned home, this mother stopped breast-feeding.

The social context for the belief in inadequate milk is illustrated in prospective studies (Sjolin *et al.* 1979). Wylie and Verber (1994) found no weight gain difference between babies of mothers who ended breast-feeding and those who did not. Erroneous beliefs about milk supply are illustrated by the following example.

> A mother was told by her mother that her softer breasts meant there was no milk for her baby any more. She began to wean but missed breast-feeding so much that she contacted a breast-feeding counsellor who explained that the breasts do not feel so full as feeding progresses. She returned to breast-feeding.

Research suggests that only 1% of women cannot produce enough milk (Akre 1989), and even malnourished women can sustain breast-feeding (Prentice and Prentice 1988). Cross-species knowledge supports the normality of frequent feeding, as do cross-cultural studies (Jelliffe and Jelliffe 1978; Widdowson 1981). Such knowledge was one strategy in a successful counselling skills support programme for women who wished to breast-feed (Jenner 1988).

Failure to thrive

A clinic in Bristol dealing with a wide range of breast-feeding concerns found that simple advice and support-based understanding and application of the basic mechanisms outlined above helped in around 80% of cases (Renfrew *et al.* 1999).

Psychological issues for the mother and baby

Some women do not enjoy breast-feeding, finding it a chore, irritant or repellent. Raphael-Leff posits a continuum of behaviours between that of 'facilitators', who are baby centred in their mothering style, and 'regulators', who prefer to have a routine-centred life into which the baby must fit (Raphael-Leff 1993). The effect on women who find breast-feeding attractive but feel they must abandon it can be devastating. Very little is known about the effect on the mother or baby of pressure towards continuing breast-feeding, where this is a negative experience.

There is a large body of research on the influences on women choosing different feeding methods, some attempting a typology of women who are likely to breast-feed. There is less interest in the effect of breast-feeding on women's emotional well being. Researchers who found that women who did not intend to breast-feed produced less milk did so at a time when iatrogenic interventions were universal. It may have been that mothers wishing to breast-feed gave extra or longer feeds or fed for longer, while those who were less enthusiastic obeyed time rules (Newton and Newton 1967). A small-scale study of low-income women in America found that the ones who succeeded in breast-feeding felt empowered by the experience (Locklin and Nabor 1993). A more women-centred research agenda would be helpful in this area.

In post-natal depression, the mother's long-term aims need to be considered. While family and health professionals may wish to rescue the mother from the demands of a baby, she may feel it is the only part of mothering she can do well, and so contraindicated drugs should be avoided. Where a mother wishes to continue breast-feeding, it should not be assumed that all antidepressants will affect the baby negatively or that drug therapy is the only form of treatment. Further research is needed in this field.

The implications on the mother–baby relationship for successful and unsuccessful breast-feeding, in the mother's terms, are many. The breast-fed baby is comparatively autonomous, e.g. *taking* the breast rather than *being given* the bottle, and finishing feeds when sated rather than when the required amount is transferred (Wright 1988). Many women find the apparently irrational and unpredictable needs of a baby intolerable and seek to solve this by offering bottles to extend inter-feed periods or to attempt lengthening intervals between feeds.

Effective help

A problem may lie at any (or many) point(s) on a physical–psychosocial continuum. The experience of feeling 'drained' may be to do with low blood sugar after several feeds with no food intake, a normal reaction to prolactin in the bloodstream or a learned response in a culture with low confidence in breast-feeding. It is known that the mother's access to support and information is more important to the alleviation than the severity of problems (Houston 1984).

Breast-feeding has become increasingly medicalised. Not all concerns respond to a diagnostic and prescriptive model but may be helped by the use of counselling skills with research-based information (Jenner 1988). Awareness of the cultural messages reaching mothers about concerns (e.g the fragility of milk supply) and the control of women's body fluids in our society is needed.

All the required helping skills are not necessarily found in one person or profession. Help may best be delivered by members of a team, with for example a paediatrician to see if the baby is well, and a midwife or breast-feeding counsellor to see if the mother and baby together are enabling effective feeding and to offer time. Conflict is avoided by good communication, with the mother's consent.

The use of basic counselling skills may provide a helpful model for intervention in this holistic area.

- Listening for personal and cultural meanings with minimal intervention and reflection allows a mother to explore her interpretation of events.
- Non-judgemental approaches allow parents to express their feelings without condemnation, reassurance or instant problem solving.
- Conveying helpful attitudes, e.g. that breast-feeding is a possibility for most women but that no one will force the mother to continue.
- Open questions help parents to keep control of the agenda, especially those that find out the mother's intentions, short and long term.
- Avoiding advice – finding out the mother's theories and what previous advice has been given and then offering suggestions and information offers parents increased control rather than adding another set of instructions and so another person to please.
- Exploring the psychosocial context – what are other people saying to her, explicitly or implicitly, now and in the past?
- Exploring the nature of the initiation of breast-feeding and its meaning to the mother.
- Avoiding physical handling of mother and baby unless by request, so as to encourage independence and understanding for the future.
- Referring to others with appropriate skills offers a range of help.

Conclusion

Increasing biomedical emphasis has highlighted breast milk as perfectly responsive to each baby's needs and capable of producing both general and specific protection against disease. Health professionals are coming to understand their role in promoting the possibility of maternal feeding as a better option for the baby, and for the mother, who also enjoys considerable health gains by breast-feeding (Standing Committee on Nutrition of the British Paediatric Association 1994). Not all professionals are yet equipped to offer sufficiently informed help, and there is a need to know where to go for expertise.

Women who do not wish or feel unable to initiate or sustain this 'choice' can easily be stigmatised. What is easily lost sight of is the psychosocial reality of day-to-day feeding. All the roles of eating and drinking – from relief from hunger and thirst, nourishment for health and hydration, to stimulus and comfort, relief of boredom and social interaction – influence the complex breast-feeding relationship, sometimes to the amazement of parents. Satisfying a baby's many needs during feeding while placating expectations of significant others and wider society often proves a difficult task for mothers when these are so often in opposition.

Feeding and comforting the newborn takes a large proportion of the new parent's day and night. With little possibility for antenatal practice or visualisation and the invisibility of breast-feeding in most Western cultures, mothers and fathers can have little understanding of the unique demands made on them at this time. Listening to the long-term aims of the mother in the context of her social and cultural setting is essential as part of the helping process in any breast-feeding crisis or concern.

Little is known of the long-term effects of initial breast-feeding difficulties on later feeding problems. In whatever way breast-feeding ends, some mothers appear relieved to lose sole responsibility for their child's nutrition, while others remain or become anxious. It is clear that issues such as autonomy, conflict, unmet expectations and satisfaction are already present in early feeding interactions and that unresolved concerns might usefully be revisited in a therapeutic setting.

References

Akre J (1989) (ed) *Infant Feeding: the physiological basis.* World Health Organisation, Geneva.

Bam-Yam NB and Darby L (1997) Fathers and breastfeeding: a review of the literature. *Journal of Human Lactation.* **13**(1): 45–50.

Barnes J, Leggett J and Durham T (1993) Breastfeeders versus bottlefeeders: differences in femininity perceptions. *Maternal–Child Nursing Journal.* **21**(1): 15–19.

British Association of Perinatal Medicine *et al.* (1997) *Hypoglycaemia of the Newborn.* National Childbirth Trust, London.

de Carvalho M, Hall M and Harvey D (1981) Effects of water supplementation on physiological jaundice in breast-fed babies. *Archives of Diseases in Childhood.* **56**(7): 568–9.

de Chateau P, Homberg H, Jakobsson K and Winberg J (1977) A study of factors promoting and inhibiting lactation. *Developmental Medicine and Child Neurology.* **19**: 575–84.

Deutsch H (1945) *The Psychology of Women, vol 2, Motherhood.* Grune and Stratton, New York.

Drewett B and Young B (1998) Methods for the analysis of feeding behaviour in infancy: sucklings. *Journal of Reproductive and Infant Psychology.* **16**: 9–26.

Evans K, Evans R and Simmer K (1995) Effect of the method of breast feeding on breast engorgement, mastitis and infantile colic. *Acta Paediatrica.* **84**(8): 849–52.

Foster K, Lader D and Cheesbrough S (1997) *Infant Feeding 1995.* HMSO, London.

Green JM, Goupland VA and Kitzinger J (1988) *Great Expectations.* Child Care and Development Group, University of Cambridge.

Hewat RJ and Ellis DJ (1986) Similarities and differences between women who breastfeed for short and long duration. *Midwifery.* **2**: 37–43.

Hin Mang-U, Nyant-Nyant-Wai, Myo-Khin, Mu-Mu-Khin, Tin-U and Thane-Toe (1985) Effect on clinical outcome of breast-feeding during acute diarrhoea. *British Medical Journal.* **290**: 587–9.

Houston MJ (1984) Home support for the breast-feeding mother. In: MJ Houston (ed) *Maternal and Infant Health Care: recent advances in nursing.* Churchill Livingstone, London.

Howie PW, Forsyth JS, Ogston SA, Clark A and Florey C du V (1989) Protective effect of breast feeding against infection. *British Medical Journal.* **300**: 11–16.

Hytten FE (1954) Clinical and chemical studies in human lactation. *British Medical Jounal.* **1**: 175–82.

Jelliffe DB and Jelliffe EFP (1978) *Human Milk in the Modern World.* Oxford University Press, Oxford.

Jenner S (1988) The influence of additional information, advice and support on the success of breast feeding in working class primiparas. *Child: Care, Health and Development.* **14**: 319–28.

Locklin MP and Nabor SJ (1993) Does breast-feeding empower women? Insights from a select group of educated, low-income, minority women. *Birth.* **20**: 30–5.

Manning M (1997) *Bounty BabyCare Guide.* Bounty Services Ltd, Norfolk.

Morbacher N and Stock J (1991) *The Breast-feeding Answerbook.* La Leche League International, Illinois.

Newton M and Newton N (1967) Psychologic aspects of lactation. *New England Journal of Medicine.* **277**(22): 1179–88.

Prentice AM and Prentice A (1988) Energy cost of lactation. *Annual Review of Nutrition.* **8**: 63–79.

Rajan L (1994) The impact of obstetric procedures and algesia/anaesthesia during labour and delivery on breast-feeding. *Midwifery.* **10**: 87–103.

Raphael-Leff J (1993) *Pregnancy: the inside story.* Sheldon Press, London.

Renfrew MJ, McGill HR and Woolridge M (1999) *Enabling Women to Breastfeed.* The Stationery Office, London (in press).

Righard L and Alade MO (1990) Effect of delivery room routines on success of first breastfeed. *Lancet.* **336**: 1105–7.

Royal College of Midwives (1991) *Successful Breastfeeding.* Churchill Livingstone, London.

Sjolin S, Hofvander Y and Hillervik C (1979) A prospective study of individual course of breastfeeding. *Acta Paediatrica Scandinavica.* **68**: 521–9.

Smale OM (1996) Women's breastfeeding. PhD thesis, University of Bradford.

Standing Committee on Nutrition of the British Paediatric Association (1994) Is breast-feeding beneficial in the UK? *Archives of Diseases in Childhood.* **71**: 376–80.

Taylor L and Littlewood J (1994) *The Breastfeeding Experiences of Mothers with Premature and Full-term Infants.* Report prepared for the National Childbirth Trust by Women and Welfare Research. Department of Social Sciences, Loughborough University.

Tew MA (1990) *Safer Childbirth? A Critical History of Maternity Care.* Chapman and Hall, London.

White A, Freeth S and O'Brien M (1992) *Infant Feeding 1990.* HMSO, London.

Widdowson EM (1981) *Feeding the Newborn Mammal.* Carolina biology reader 112. Carolina Biological Supply Company, Burlington, North Carolina.

Woolridge MW and Fisher C (1988) Colic, 'overfeeding' and symptoms of lactose malabsorption in the breast-fed baby: a possible artifact of feed management? *Lancet.* **2**: 382–4.

Woolridge MW, Baum JD and Drewett RF (1980) Effect of a traditional and of a new nipple shield on sucking patterns and milk flow. *Early Human Development.* **4**(4): 357–64.

Wright P (1988) Learning experiences during feeding behaviour during infancy. *Journal of Psychosomatic Research.* **32**(6): 613–19.

Wylie J and Verber IJ (1994) Why women fail to breastfeed: a prospective study from booking to 28 days post-partum. *International Journal of Human Nutrition and Dietetics.* **7**: 115–20.

Further reading

Culley P, Milan P, Roginski C, Waterhouse J and Wood B (1979) Are breast-fed babies still getting a raw deal in hospital? *British Medical Journal.* **6195**(2): 891–3.

Henly SJ, Anderson CM, Avery MD, Hills-Bonczyk SG, Potter S and Duckett LJ (1995) Anemia and insufficient milk in first-time mothers. *Birth: Issues in Perinatal Care and Education.* **22**(2): 87–92.

Henschel D (1996) *Breast-feeding: a guide for midwives.* Books for Midwives Press, Hale.

Lang S (1997) *Breast-feeding Special Care Babies.* Baillière Tindall, London.

Marmet C, Shell E and Marmet R (1990) Neonatal frenotomy may be necessary to correct breast-feeding problems. *Journal of Human Lactation.* **6**(3): 117–21.

Mathur GP, Chitranshi S, Mathur S, Singh SB and Bhalla M (1992) Lactation failure. *Indian Pediatrics.* **29**(12): 1541–4.

McIntosh J (1985) Barriers to breast feeding: choice of feeding method in a sample of working class primaparae. *Midwifery.* **1**: 213–24.

Renfrew MJ (1989) Positioning the baby at the breast: more than a visual skill. *Journal of Human Lactation.* **5**(1): 13–15.

Righard L and Alade MO (1992) Sucking technique and its effect on success of breastfeeding. *Birth.* **19**(4): 185–9.

CHAPTER 9

The management of selective eating in young children

Jo Douglas

Introduction

Selective eating or faddiness is a common behavioural problem in young children. It is often transient and short-lived, with food preferences altering every few weeks or lasting for a few months at most. In some children it becomes a severe and chronic problem which affects their health, socialisation and ability to mix with peers. They refuse to go to parties, are unable to eat out socially and are extremely rigid about the conditions under which they will eat and what they will eat.

Children who are severe selective eaters fall into two major categories. Children in the first category may drink excessive quantities of milk or squash, which reduces their appetite and consequently reduces the range of food they are prepared to eat. They have developed a habit pattern and mistake the signal of hunger for that of thirst. These children frequently are highly dependent on bottles and gain a lot of comfort and satisfaction from sucking. The second group of severely selective children are those who tend to eat a highly restricted range of food, which usually falls into the carbohydrate range, i.e. crisps, biscuits, bread, cereal and chips, but they will also frequently drink milk or eat fromage frais, which maintains a balance in their diet. The most frequently refused foods are fruit, vegetables, pulses, meat and fish. Some eat an excessive amount of sweets and chocolate, which can significantly harm their teeth.

Prevalence of selective eating in pre-school children

In a large retrospective population study, 4% of five-year-olds were described as being 'faddy' by their parents. There was an equal prevalence in boys and girls. Thirty percent of the faddy eaters had feeding problems as a baby (Butler and Golding 1986). Richman *et al.* (1982) found that 12% of three-year-olds were faddy eaters, as identified on the Behaviour Screening Questionnaire. When the rate of faddy eating was examined in a group of children defined as having behaviour problems this percentage increased to 31%.

Severe selective eating in young children is not well described in the literature. It is often included in general samples of children treated as food refusers. Douglas and Bryon (1996) indicate that severe selective eating was present in a third of their sample of young children with severe eating problems, but the symptom was not a definitive classification as some of the same children also had comorbid features of severe problems with quantity or texture of food for their age. Timimi *et al.* (1997) describe selective eating in two age ranges of children: those attending a pre-school feeding programme and those referred to an eating disorder programme for young adolescents. Werle *et al.* (1993) describe the treatment of three chronic food-refusing children, two of whom are selective eaters while the third has difficulties with eating age-appropriate textures of food, where a home-based behavioural programme was successfully implemented. Archer and Szatmari (1990) describe a case study of food aversion which had elements of selective eating; Singer *et al.* (1992) describe three boys with food phobias one of whom is a selective eater.

Chatoor (1997) has attempted to provide a classification of feeding disorders and describes extreme food selectivity as food refusal. She sees this as a disorder of separation with onset between six months and three years of age during the transition to self-feeding. There is variable food refusal, which is often situational. The child frequently bargains about food and has conflicts about eating with the parents, who are extremely anxious about the food refusal. She sees this problem developing from conflicts in autonomy and control and by lack of appropriate limit setting by the parents.

Other attempts to classify eating problems in young children have identified the problem with range of food as compared to problems with quantity and texture that some young children show (Douglas 1995a,b).

Aetiology of selective eating

In a paediatrically based feeding programme for children under the age of seven years at Great Ormond Street, severe selective eating is one of the referral conditions (Douglas and Bryon 1996). Clinical experience has indicated that many of these children may be highly selective over long periods in early childhood and yet can maintain reasonable weights as they eat large quantities of foods that they prefer or supplement their diet by drinking large quantities of milk.

These children often present as being phobic of their non-preferred food. If it is presented to them they may physically shake and cry or become aggressive and confrontational in an effort to avoid it. They appear to feel extremely anxious about food. This heightened state of arousal also affects other eating-related behaviours. These children are often reported to be meticulous about the presentation of food (Timimi *et al.* 1997). They may become upset if the food touches other food on the same plate, demand for different foods to be placed on separate plates, are specific about brands of food or particular flavours they will eat, or demand that it is cut in a particular way. They may be concerned about food or mess on their fingers. They may eat certain foods only in certain places or demand that the parent takes their 'home' food or own utensils whenever they go out.

This 'obsessional' behaviour can affect other areas of behavioural development and the child can show compulsive traits, e.g. rituals about falling asleep, excessive tidiness, concern about clothes matching or shoelaces being tied exactly the same. They may have difficulties with separation and with socialisation at nursery or school. It is possible that there is a continuum of severity of selective eating, ranging from the erratic food faddiness of pre-school children through the severely selective children to children with severe difficulties with socialisation, e.g. semantic pragmatic disorder and autism. Many of the features seen in the severely selective child are present in this more severe end of the spectrum of developmental disorder.

For example, Laurie, aged four years, had been diagnosed with semantic pragmatic disorder, but he had started to speak in the previous six months and could communicate reasonably at assessment. He had a significant number of behaviour problems, including obsessional and repetitive play with specific toys, sleeping difficulties and severe tantrums twice a day. The parents, with behavioural management advice, had been able to set clear limits for his behaviour and resolved the night waking. His diet had become progressively restricted by the age of 18 months of age. At assessment he would eat only 'smiley face' potato shapes, bananas and milk, and his weight was between the 75th and 90th percentiles. He was extremely avoidant of any other food and vehemently refused to try new foods.

It is not clear why these children become severely selective eaters, although certain hypotheses can be considered and revealed through the assessment process. Parents frequently report early onset under the age of two years in pre-school children. Most of this age group show onset of symptomatology at the introduction of lumpy stage 2 baby foods, although it can appear earlier with infants of three months of age rejecting different tastes of stage 1 purées. Breast- or bottle-feeding usually presented no problems. Parents can often identify events that triggered the start of the problem, e.g. choking on a specific food or after a bout of diarrhoea and vomiting. Some children show onset after they have accepted solid and finger foods and they become progressively more selective over time. They will gag, choke and retch on non-preferred food and will refuse to swallow it.

In a sample of 34 children diagnosed as selective eaters in the Great Ormond Street Feeding Programme, 100% of the children had started to be selective by the age of two years, 85% by the age of one year and 47% by six months of age. The transition to the lumpier stage 2 baby food had created a problem for most of the children.

Assessment of the problem

A detailed account of the date of onset of the problem, the medical history and the eating history of the child is an essential feature of assessment (see Chapter 3). There is usually no concern about their physical health, although some children who drink excessively large amounts of sugary fruit squash or eat large quantities of chocolate may have dental caries. For example, Jack, aged five years, had 15 teeth removed due to severe dental caries as his diet consisted of chocolate and milk.

Some children may have a history of repeated ENT problems and enlarged tonsils while others may show some sensitivity to dairy products, but in general the range of medical problems identified in these children is insignificant compared to those of general referrals to a paediatric feeding programme.

Observation of a meal time with the parents will provide information about the behaviour patterns and how they are being maintained. Observation of how the child reacts to non-preferred foods being on their plate will often provide clear guidance as to how the existing pattern of behaviour has become entrenched. Children frequently are uncooperative, will not come to the table or sit down, they push the plate away, whine and moan, or cry and become upset. The parents may give in very quickly if they are unable to cope with the child's distress, they may be unable to get the child even to come and sit at the table and they may rapidly offer a preferred alternative food.

For example, Jamie aged four years refused to sit down and eat the crisps that were on his plate with other food. The parents requested that the packet of crisps be brought in to show him that they were his preferred brand and he agreed to eat some tipped out of the packet in front of him. He then demanded that the parents shut their eyes while he ate the first one and sat on the floor under the table to do so. Once he had tasted the first crisp he accepted that they were his type of crisp and proceeded to eat the rest perfectly well and even took the original ones from the main plate of food.

The child's distress and protestations will suddenly disappear when the preferred food is offered. The child may eat it rapidly in large mouthfuls as they feel confident and relieved. They frequently ask for more. But some children will nibble around the edges of even their preferred food and eat relatively slowly. Observing these differences in eating style is important for the development of a hypothesis about how to treat the child. Children who nibble could be considered to have a mild oral-motor dysfunction and find that they prefer the bite–dissolve foods that this easy range of carbohydrates provides.

Parents may also have very different styles of coping with the child, one often being more lenient and compliant than the other. Parents may disregard each other's attempts to encourage the child to eat, undermine the actions of the other parent or be more impatient and less tolerant than the other. They may be very positive with the child encouraging them to try food, but they often ask questions rather than make statements or give clear instructions about what is expected and leave themselves open to a clear refusal. The tentative nature of the request to try a food only reinforces the child's power in the situation. Some parents will not comment if their child does try a new food for fear of making too big an issue out of it, of making the child embarrassed or of putting him or her off repeating the attempt. In general the parents are extremely anxious about the child's food refusal and may try excessively to encourage the child to eat, or alternatively give the child anything that he or she wants to eat at any time.

The hypotheses about aetiology fall into four main groups.

- Anxiety about food has been generated in the child by previous aversive experiences with allergic reactions or difficulties with swallowing lumpy food due to medical problems, e.g. recurrent enlarged tonsils.
- An 'obsessional' or anxious personality style in the child where a choking incident is amplified by the child's predisposition to be anxious.
- Anxiety generated in parents, which leads them to restrict the types of foods they offer their child and a consequent lack of ability to confront the child about the range of food that he or she is eating.
- Parental management style that allows the child to take control and make choices for themselves with poor limit setting and poor boundaries.

Treatment approaches

When families attend for treatment there are several major characteristics that the clinician should take into account.

- The parents have a long experience of their child not eating a wide range of foods and have already accommodated to this.
- The parents will have tried a wide range of methods to try and encourage their child to eat a wider range and feel helpless and impotent.

- The parents are usually upset about other people's comments that the child needs a good slap, should be starved or that anyone can get a child to eat, but feel helpless.
- The parents' anxiety about maintaining the child's weight is managed by giving the child a lot of the limited range of food he or she will eat.
- Most parents are concerned that they might have caused the problem in some way.
- The child is used to getting his or her own way about what he or she eats and how he or she eats.
- The child is very strong willed.
- The child is very fearful of new foods and does not want to try them.
- The child does not know why he or she cannot eat a wide range of foods and probably does not want to change.
- The child has a repertoire of food-avoidant behaviours that are effective in the family.
- The child and the family do not know how to change the existing state of affairs.

Recognition, acceptance and reassurance about the problem are important. Parents' concerns need to be taken seriously. Most of these children are not unwell, are not failing to thrive and the problem is really a social and psychological one. Parents often say that they owe it to their child to try and solve the problem and are usually very motivated for treatment. They worry about long-term outcome and do not want to be blamed later by their child because he or she is still on a restricted diet.

A behavioural management approach to treatment has been demonstrated to be of value. Taking a behavioural perspective it is possible to identify both classical and operant conditioning experiences that may have influenced the development of the child's selective eating. Classical conditioning will have occurred when the child's experience of eating has been paired repeatedly with an unpleasant experience, perhaps force, pain, nausea or fear. Operant conditioning will have occurred when the child's difficult behaviour has resulted in parents giving in to his or her demands or providing only preferred foods. Treatment strategies therefore need to take into account stimulus control issues, i.e. events or stimuli that precede the intake of food and elicit fear reactions, as well as contingent events aimed at reinforcing the acceptance of new foods.

Parents, similarly, have a learning history with their child and have evolved a method of keeping their anxiety as low as possible. Patterson's (1982) coercive hypothesis of family functioning is a useful explanatory model (Figure 9.1). The mother rapidly learns not to offer food the child does not like. She reduces the behavioural disturbance, the emotional upset and her concern about adequate nutritional intake by offering the child his or her

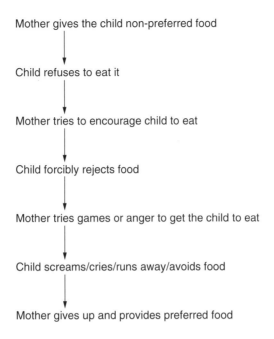

Mother gives the child non-preferred food

↓

Child refuses to eat it

↓

Mother tries to encourage child to eat

↓

Child forcibly rejects food

↓

Mother tries games or anger to get the child to eat

↓

Child screams/cries/runs away/avoids food

↓

Mother gives up and provides preferred food

Figure 9.1: Patterson's coercive hypothesis of family functioning.

preferred foods. The child equally learns that if he or she causes enough disruption and upset then he or she will get his or her own way.

The focus of treatment is at several levels:

- to build up the child's confidence and self-esteem about trying new foods
- to desensitise the child's fear of new food and change
- to enable the parents to set clear limits for their child and to expect compliance
- to introduce a graded system of introduction of new foods including texture, range and quantity
- to increase the range of foods eaten in a systematic manner
- to reinforce the child's success at trying new foods
- to maintain the child's weight and growth.

If the child is old enough or has sufficient language it is often helpful to gauge his or her level of motivation for change by enquiring directly. Some will indicate that they would like to be able to eat some other foods some day, others will give a complete denial or even refuse to talk about the issue. The child will usually be happy to talk about the range of foods that he or she can eat and this can be confirmed by the parents. A list of preferred foods is important in planning the changes that need to take place.

Treatment plan

Planning treatment requires full cooperation and motivation from the parents as they need to apply the plan on a regular basis at home two or three times a day at meal times. They need to acknowledge that it is going to be a long, slow process of change that will require consistency and firmness of resolve. The child will be reluctant to change and requires help to face up to the challenge in small, manageable steps.

Stimulus control methods to reduce fear of new food by desensitisation prior to the child learning to put a new food into his or her mouth may be necessary if the child is extremely anxious or the parents are unable to cope with the child's level of resistance. A systematic plan of initially just touching the new food, putting it to lips, kissing it, licking it, sucking it and then putting it in his or her mouth over several days or weeks can be successful. This 'shaping' procedure helps the child learn all of the necessary skills prior to eating.

Once the child has become less fearful then the next stages of change are as follows:

1 Choose a new, non-preferred food to taste that is close to the range that the child already eats easily, e.g. a new type of bread, or biscuit, or a new flavour of crisp.
2 Expect the child to eat a tiny piece or crumb of the new food (approximately half a centimetre in size) at each meal and snack time before they are allowed to eat the preferred food or drink.
3 Offer the same new food for four days before changing to a new one.
4 Increase the size of the piece of the new food on successive presentations once the child starts to eat it without distress.
5 Develop a reward programme associated with success, e.g. an Eat Up book where the child sticks in a picture or labels of food that he or she can eat and has tasted, or sticker charts for trying a new food.
6 Introduce new foods outside the carbohydrate range once the child has accepted the new pattern.

The aim is for the parents to be successful in instructing the child in what to do. Having a clear expectation and goal that is within the ability of the child to achieve is vital. Both the parent and the child need to feel success: the parents by realising that they can set limits for their child and achieve compliance; the child for having managed a new skill. Some children are very fearful of change and require resolute and firm control from their parents. Others will need to learn skills to cope orally with the new food, putting larger amounts in their mouths, learning to chew and move food around their mouths.

The success of the changes achieved depends on the parents' ability to set limits and establish boundaries about food. It is often a long and slow struggle to achieve change with the child readily reverting to preferred foods if given a chance. It is rare for a child to be able to eat all types of food at the end of treatment, i.e. to sit down to a roast dinner of meat and two vegetables, but they are usually able to eat a wider range of children's-type foods, including some vegetables and other forms of protein such as fish fingers, chicken fingers, sandwiches with different fillings, and cheese. They are not so confined by brand names and eat a wider range of foods than they had previously eaten, e.g. all different types of biscuits, crisps and breakfast cereals. The increase in range of foods eaten makes it easier for them to eat socially at friends' houses or to go out for a meal with their family.

Case study 1

David was eating Weetabix with hot milk for three meals a day at age five years. In addition he would eat McCoys or Walkers crisps, frozen chips, a couple of teaspoons of spaghetti hoops, sandwiches without filling, smooth yoghurt, milk chocolate, jelly or gum sweets and Rolos. His eating problem had started when lumpy foods had been introduced. He would gag, choke and vomit on the lumpy textures. In addition his range of food dramatically reduced at the age of 2.5 years when his sister was born.

The aim of treatment was for meal times to become calmer and less aversive, and for the parents to be able to set expectations about what David should eat and the quantity he should eat. The family chose the reinforcer to be 15 minutes on the computer with father after having tried a new food, but if he made a scene for the reward to be withdrawn without anger or reproach. He was expected to eat a tiny amount of the new food before his preferred food. At times he would take over an hour to try the speck of new food, but his parents persevered and kept to their plan despite the strain. David gradually began to try more foods and a star chart was introduced where he could earn one star for eating a particular size of a new food and one for eating it in a set time limit. Gradually two new foods were introduced every other day and the resistance to meal times reduced.

About halfway through the programme there was a slight setback as David started to store food in his mouth. His parents' expectations had accelerated slightly faster than David's ability to change. His father started to shout at him for slow chewing and he was starting to receive more attention for bad behaviour than appropriate behaviour at the table. The chart system was modified to give him a silver star for eating half of the amount in a certain time and a gold star for finishing his plate in the agreed time. His mother also started a game of counting to swallow a food. By the end of treatment (12 attendances) David was starting to ask for new foods and was willing to try. The range of foods he was eating had increased to include sausages, fish fingers, spaghetti bolognese, rice, pasta and biscuits.

Case study 2

Sam, aged seven years, was referred as he was eating only liquidised foods prepared by his mother in her food blender, plus particular brands of biscuits, yoghurt and crisps. His problem had started at the age of seven months when he had choked on a rusk. He had demonstrated significant oral motor delay and gagged when solid food was placed in his mouth from that time. Sam also had a moderate developmental delay but his language was in keeping with his other developmental skills. He disliked mess on his hands and was reluctant to touch food. His weight was in the average range.

The treatment plan aims were:

- to encourage him to touch foods by handling food at home, putting fruit and vegetables into bags in the supermarket, giving his hamster pieces of lettuce and cucumber
- to thicken the texture of the blended food by adding more potato and reducing the liquid content
- to introduce new brands of preferred foods, i.e. biscuits and crisps, and avoid buying his preferred brands
- to introduce tiny portions of new foods
- to stop him gagging and choking by clear instruction
- to use an Eat Up book as a reward
- to increase his tolerance to new textures of food.

Sam was extremely avoidant of new foods, would argue and refuse to eat. Initially, to encourage him to eat some thickened purée it was necessary to offer a crisp as a reinforcer for each mouthful. His mother decided early on that if he gagged and tried to vomit she would make him eat an extra spoonful. This had the effect of stopping the gagging rapidly. Gradually over the course of 10 sessions Sam managed to learn to eat small quantities of a variety of foods. His mother stopped liquidising his food after six sessions, by which time he had started to eat small quantities of soft food, e.g. Dairylea, spaghetti hoops, toast and cooked carrots. His pattern of eating the more solid foods was one of nibbling small pieces and chewing them thoroughly before swallowing, which made the meal times very prolonged.

His mother was extremely committed and persevered with each new stage of change. She acknowledged the immense amount of effort it took to encourage change in Sam. By the end of the programme Sam could eat a small amount of a wide range of foods, including fish fingers, sausages, chips, baked beans and pasta. He was still needing approximately half of his calorie intake from his preferred range of food after having eaten the new range.

At follow-up five years later, at the age of 12 years, he was still eating a variety of food and the good progress had been maintained and extended. His mother still had to be firm about varying his range so that he does not become fixed on to any one type of food. He had made little further progress with vegetables and would still gag if given them.

Prognosis and outcome

A simple telephone follow-up of seven children, referred for severe and chronic selective eating, three years after completing the treatment programme in the Great Ormond Street Hospital Feeding Programme revealed that three children had totally normal diets, three children were the same as they were at the end of treatment and had not extended their range of foods further, while one child was eating a more limited range than he had at the end of treatment. It is clear that these children can extend their range of foods with behavioural management techniques but it requires great effort and commitment from the parents to carry out the treatment programme and then to carry it on after leaving the treatment programme.

The natural outcome of severe selective eating in early childhood has not been documented. From clinical experience it is clear that many of these children continue their selective eating throughout childhood and some into adult life but the epidemiology of this problem is not known. Anecdotal evidence and retrospective information from adults who were selective eaters as children point to the possibility of the child or adolescent deciding to extend their range of foods at a significant life change, e.g. starting secondary school, going out on the first date, leaving home or getting married. Severe selective eating exists in the adult population but it is not clear whether this originated in early childhood or infancy. A long-term follow-up study would be valuable to document the progress of these children.

It is possible that there may be a comorbid association with obsessional and ritualistic behaviour and that there may be continuity with the selective eating seen in many children with autistic spectrum disorders. Children who fall into the autistic spectrum disorder range are much more difficult to treat, so it may be possible to see a continuum of severity and prognosis dependent on the presence of comorbid features.

References

Archer LA and Szatmari P (1990) Assessment and treatment of food aversion in a four year old boy: a multidimensional approach. *Canadian Journal of Psychiatry.* **35**: 501–5.

Butler NR and Golding J (eds) (1986) *From Birth to Five. A Study of the Health and Behaviour of Britain's Five Year Olds.* Pergamon Press, London.

Chatoor I (1997) Feeding disorders of infants and toddlers. In: JD Noshpitz (ed) *Handbook of Child and Adolescent Psychiatry, vol. 1. Infants and Pre-schoolers: development and syndromes* S Greenspan, S Wieder and J Osofsky (eds). John Wiley and Sons, New York.

Douglas JE (1995a) Behavioural eating disorders in young children. *Current Paediatrics.* **5**: 39–42.

Douglas JE (1995b) Behavioural eating problems in young children In: P Davies (ed) *Nutrition in Child Health.* Royal College of Physicians, BPA, London.

Douglas JE and Bryon M (1996) Interview data on severe behavioural eating difficulties in young children. *Archives of Diseases in Childhood.* **75**: 304–8.

Patterson GR (1982) *Coercive Family Process: a social learning approach.* Castalia, Eugene, Oregon.

Richman N, Stephenson J and Graham PJ (1982) *Pre-school to School. A Behavioural Study.* Academic Press, London.

Singer LT, Ambuel B, Wade S and Jaffe AC (1992) Cognitive-behavioural treatment of health impairing food phobias in children. *Journal of the American Academy of Child and Adolescent Psychiatry.* **31**: 847–52.

Timimi S, Douglas J and Tsiftsopoulou K (1997) Selective eaters: a retrospective case note study. *Child: Care, Health and Development.* **23**: 265–78.

Werle MA, Murphy TB and Budd KS (1993) Treating chronic food refusal in young children: home based parent training. *Journal of Applied Behaviour Analysis.* **26**: 421–33.

CHAPTER 10

Assessing feeding in children with neurological problems

Sheena Reilly, Alison Wisbeach and Lucinda Carr

Introduction

This chapter focuses on the assessment of feeding in children with neurological problems where there is a readily identifiable organic component. It takes an integrationist perspective, highlighting the collaborative working of speech and language therapy, occupational therapy and paediatric neurology. Much of the chapter is concerned with dysphagia, a condition common to many children with neurological impairment. It presents an overview of the characteristics and consequences of dysphagia, before going on to consider multidisciplinary assessment procedures.

The characteristics and prevalence of dysphagia

The term 'dysphagia' is used to describe any disorder of swallowing which occurs in the oral, pharyngeal and/or oesophageal stages of deglutition. Subsumed in this definition are problems with positioning food in the mouth and in oral movements, including suckling, sucking and chewing. The anatomical and physiological substrates of dysphagia in children with neurological problems are complex. In the child with multiple disability, disorders of swallowing, or dysphagia, are rarely the presenting feature. Similarly, dysphagia in children with neurological problems rarely arises from one single cause. The aetiology is likely to be multifactorial and may involve the whole digestive tract (*see* Figure 10.1). It is important to consider the emotional and psychological aspects of eating and drinking, since many problems present as a combination of organic and non-organic factors. Aetiological factors include gross motor difficulties, problems of the oral,

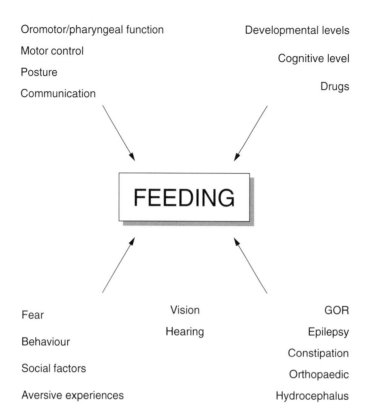

Figure 10.1: Factors that may affect feeding the child with neurological impairment.

pharyngeal and oesophageal stages and the process of elimination. Equally important contributory factors such as communication and the preparatory stage of feeding should be considered.

There is no doubt that dysphagia is a common but under-recognised problem, particularly in the child with four-limb involvement. Clinicians should not forget that dysphagia is also seen in other types of cerebral palsy and in a number of less common conditions, such as inborn errors of metabolism (particularly glutaric aciduria), neurodegenerative conditions (such as Leigh's disease) and some acquired conditions (such as traumatic brain injury). Although this chapter focuses on the child with cerebral palsy, the basic principles of assessment and management, once established, are readily transferable between groups of children with neurological problems with different aetiologies.

Dysphagia may occur as part of a congenital or an acquired condition. It is a particular feature of a number of genetic disorders/syndromes and of certain types of cerebral palsy. Dysphagia may also arise from other cerebral insults such as trauma, infection, metabolic disease and neurodegenerative disorders.

The nature of the resulting problems may be structural, neuromuscular or functional, or indeed a combination of all three.

The exact prevalence of dysphagia in the majority of syndromes/disorders is unknown. Most studies have been beset by poor methodology. Children with cerebral palsy form the largest group presenting to a tertiary dysphagia clinic (Carr *et al.* 1997) and there are a number of studies describing the nature and extent of dysphagia in this group.

The prevalence of cerebral palsy in developed countries is around two per 1000 live births (Hagberg *et al.* 1996). Numbers have remained surprisingly constant over the past 40 years. This partly reflects the antenatal aetiology of many of the cerebral palsies. Furthermore, any reduction due to improved maternal health has been offset by the increased survival of pre-term infants. As a result there has been an increase in the proportion of severely affected children (Hagberg *et al.* 1996).

The process of feeding

In understanding dysphagia, it is important to be aware of the oral-motor skills involved in the process of feeding. There are three stages involved in eating and drinking: the oral phase involves preparing the food within the oral cavity and transporting it to the back of the mouth in readiness for triggering the swallow; during the pharyngeal phase, food and liquid are moved safely through the pharynx by the swallowing process and transported into the oesophagus (oesophageal stage). Each stage must be considered individually and as an integrated function (*see* Table 10.1). Disruption to any of the three phases of swallowing can cause significant impairment of the eating and drinking process and result in dysphagia. The preceding anticipatory and preparatory stages of feeding should also be examined as they may involve subtle psychological factors.

Oral stage

In a study of pre-school children with cerebral palsy (aged between 12 and 79 months) Reilly *et al.* (1996) found that nine of the 10 children had clinically significant oral-motor dysfunction. Of this group more than a third (36.2%) had severe oral-motor impairment and these tended to be children with four-limb motor involvement, as highlighted in previous studies (Stallings *et al.* 1993).

Table 10.1: Characteristics of oral, pharyngeal and oesophageal dysphagia in children with cerebral palsy

Oral stage	Poor/absent bolus formation
	Poor/absent transportation of bolus
	Poor/absent manipulation of bolus
	Poor/absent tongue lateralisation/elevation, etc.
	Poor/absent ability to retain food/liquid bolus within oral cavity
	Poor/absent lip/jaw closure
	Premature overspill into pharynx
Pharyngeal stage	Delayed/absent swallow reflex
	Aspiration/penetration before, during, after swallow
	Incomplete clearance of food/liquid residue
	Pooling of food/liquid in valleculae or pyriform sinus
	Nasal regurgitation
	Poorly coordinated ventilatory cycle and swallowing
	Slow pharyngeal transit
	Reduced peristalsis
Oesophageal stage	Gastro-oesophageal reflux
	Oesophageal dysmotility
	Delayed gastric emptying
	Oesophagitis
	Aspiration of GOR

Pharyngeal stage

There are few studies that examine the prevalence of pharyngeal stage problems. One study found that 60% of the children assessed with a modified barium swallow were at risk of aspiration (Gisel 1992). Aspiration indicates the passage of food and/or liquid into the airway below the level of the vocal folds. This may occur before, during or after swallowing. Penetration is the passage of food/or liquid into the airway but not below the level of the vocal folds. In an audit of clinic attendees studied by Carr *et al.* (1997), 66% of the children who aspirated during a modified barium swallow were suspected to be at risk from history and clinical evaluation.

Oesophageal stage

Oesophageal stage problems are also common. Sondheimer and Morris (1979) evaluated a series of severely affected children and found that up to 75% had reported gastro-oesophageal reflux (GOR). Gastro-oesophageal reflux refers to the spontaneous return of the gastric contents into the oesophagus. Gastric contents may be refluxed into the pharynx and cause regurgitation and/or vomiting. Similarly, Carr *et al.* (1997) found that reflux was demonstrated in 86% of 49 children with cerebral palsy referred for further investigation.

Consequences

The consequences of dysphagia are widespread and range in severity. At their most extreme, they may be life threatening. The consequences are summarised below.

Failure to thrive

Direct links have been made between reduced calorie intake and poor growth in children with cerebral palsy (Thommessan *et al.* 1991). Reduced body weight, linear growth, triceps and subscapular thickness have been found in the majority of children with spastic quadriplegia (Stallings *et al.* 1993). There are a number of reasons why children with cerebral palsy have difficulty achieving an adequate nutritional intake. While adequate calories may be taken, there may be excessive loss due to vomiting and regurgitation (usually as a result of gastro-oesophageal reflux). Caloric intake may be inadequate; oral and pharyngeal function may be so poor that some children may take up to 18 times longer than normal to eat a single mouthful of food. In such cases even excessively long meal times will not compensate for the severity of the dysphagia (Gisel and Patrick 1988). Whatever the cause, the resulting malnutrition has wide-ranging effects that often go beyond physical growth. There may be neurodevelopmental consequences for psychomotor development and brain growth may be directly affected. Furthermore, there are recognised effects on the immune, skeletal and cardiovascular systems (Rosenbloom and Sullivan 1996).

Specific nutrient deficiency

Micronutrient deficiencies have been reported in children with cerebral palsy (Patrick and Gisel 1990). Disabled children are at risk of iron deficiency especially if their diets are limited to ready-prepared baby foods and prolonged use of cow's milk (Rosenbloom and Sullivan 1996).

Respiratory compromise

Recurrent aspiration in non-ambulant children with neurological disease may result in repeated respiratory tract infections and can eventually lead to chronic pulmonary disease.

Pain and discomfort

Feeding is just one potential cause of pain and discomfort in children with a neurological problem. Many children have super-added communication difficulties, making it vital to consider all the potential sources of pain and discomfort. The presence of GOR can cause pain and irritability as well as damage to the lining of the oesophagus (oesophagitis) resulting in ulceration and bleeding. Additional sources of pain include constipation (see below) and dental pain.

Constipation

Constipation is a common problem in cerebral palsy. It may be due to a number of factors, including poor fibre and fluid intake, immobility, dysmotility of the lower bowel and medication (Claydon 1996). Constipation may be painful and also lead to a decrease in appetite, deterioration in behaviour and concentration. In some children it may compromise urinary continence (Claydon 1996). Dental pain (see below) and pain from other sources (such as joint pain, particularly hips, and skin abrasions, etc.) must also be considered.

Dental problems

Both hygiene and structure may be compromised. Dental care may be limited and dental caries therefore develop in children who do not tolerate tooth brushing, cannot completely empty their mouths of food residue and cannot use their tongue to clean particles of food from the teeth or gums. Children who drool excessively are deprived of the cleansing properties of saliva. Some anti-convulsants (e.g. phenytoin) have an adverse effect on oral hygiene, resulting in gingival hyperplasia. Finally, there is an increased incidence of malocclusions (Sandler *et al.* 1974) and contractures of the temporomandibular joint have also been noted in children with spastic quadriplegia (Pelegrano *et al.* 1994).

Social effects

Meal times normally serve an important social function and this may be lost in the child with dysphagia, where the routines, timing and processes associated with feeding may be disturbed. There is no doubt that meal times are often stressful occasions for the child, the feeder and the family.

The multidisciplinary approach

In common with other children with complex feeding problems, the dysphagic child may be seen by a large number of professionals. The complexity of the difficulties that present in children with dysphagia as a result of neurological problems mean that they cannot be satisfactorily dealt with by any one professional. A multidisciplinary team approach is therefore essential to both assess and manage them appropriately and efficiently (*see* Table 10.2). In order to avoid any confusion or conflicting advice, key workers are often used to help coordinate these complex cases.

Table 10.2: Multidisciplinary team members

Stage 1	Stage 2
• Paediatrician/neurologist	• Gastroenterologist
• Speech and language therapist	• Radiologist
• Occupational therapist	• Dietician
• Psychologist	• Nurse
	• Surgeon

Assessment procedures

There are a number of areas that should be included in the interview or background to the dysphagia assessment. These are summarised below.

History

A thorough assessment should always include a detailed history. The history will naturally focus on feeding, but it is vital that information regarding other aspects of the child's development is also included as it may have particular relevance to the presenting problem. Parents do not usually mind repeating details about their child's development providing it is done sensitively and the rationale is explained. It may be distressing for parents to 'retell' details of the birth history and diagnostic process and therefore professional judgement is needed to decide when this is relevant. Table 10.3 summarises the most salient points required in the history.

Much of the background information may be available from the child's

Table 10.3: Areas to be covered in the medical and feeding history

Medical diagnosis	How/when the diagnosis was made Confirmatory tests Known associated impairments What are the child's major difficulties at present?
Neonatal history	General concerns Early feeding (methods used) Type and duration of non-oral feeding Establishing oral feeding (difficulties reported) Progression to weaning (difficulties reported) Duration of feeds Vomiting/regurgitation Intervention strategies to date
General medical history	Developmental history • drooling • motor development • hearing/vision • speech/cognitive function Past medical history • hospitalisation for significant illness • surgical procedures (orthopaedic, neurosurgical, etc.) Review of systems to include: • respiratory (cough/wheeze/chest infection) • gastrointestinal (vomiting/regurgitation) • mediastinal or abdominal pain/constipation • neurological (abnormal movements, feed-related) • general affect (behaviour/sleep, etc.) • seizures • vision and hearing
Medication	Current (anti-convulsants, laxatives, etc.) Previous trials of treatment (anti-reflux medication, etc.)
Professionals involved	Social Medical Educational
Psychosocial factors	Family structure Support mechanisms

medical notes or referral letter, but in elucidating the severity and significance of specific symptoms, more detailed information is inevitably required (*see* Table 10.4). The value of an accurate feeding history cannot be over-emphasised. Nor can it be assumed that the history as described in previous reports is accurate and complete. In some cases a detailed feeding history may never have been previously established despite the fact that it is critical in understanding the child's current difficulties. Histories are also taken by a

Table 10.4: Areas to be covered in the interview

Feeding history	
Current feeding practices	Feeding diary • typical day's intake • routines • methods (e.g. who feeds) • duration/frequency of feeds • tastes/textures Oral/non-oral feeding • ratio oral to non-oral • bolus versus continuous feeds • type of tube-feed Appetite Behaviours and responses at meal times
Feeding-related issues	Positioning • special seating • special routines/equipment/techniques • who feeds Utensils
Child health and well being	Sleeping behaviour Bowel habits Growth Respiratory symptoms
Communication	How does the child communicate? • at what level? • does he/she indicate hunger/thirst or pain/discomfort?

variety of professionals whose focus inevitably varies. Furthermore, parents may come to accept long-standing feeding abnormalities as 'normal' for their child, so that questions should be open ended where possible.

Clinical examination

The clinical examination should involve both general and specific observations:

• observation of the child
• medical and neurological examination
• postural examination, including fine motor abilities
• oral motor and pharyngeal function
• observation of a feed.

Observation of the child

The aim of the examination is twofold: first, to confirm the clinical impressions gained from the history in evaluating the physical signs, in particular oro-mandibular structure, general nutritional status, respiratory and gastro-intestinal signs; second, the examination aims to clarify the neurological difficulties and identify unrecognised problems.

Medical and neurological assessment

It is important to undertake a general medical and neurological assessment, paying attention to anthropometric status and possible signs of nutritional deficiency. Assessment may also include laboratory tests to indicate adequacy of calorie and protein intake. Other blood serum values may also be sought, depending on the child's condition.

General examination will include assessment of the respiratory system both pre- and post-feed, observing signs of respiratory distress, chest deformity and intercostal recession. The quality of the breath sounds (wheeze or crepitus) should be noted. The abdomen should be palpated to confirm any tenderness or constipation. The skeletal system should be examined regarding joint range, observing for pain on movement and noting any contractures. Spinal mobility should be checked and scoliosis noted. The neurological assessment examines for muscle tone, power and reflexes. Quality of movement and the presence of involuntary movements should be observed. Cranial nerves and bulbar function should be evaluated.

Postural examination

Postural stability is critical to the child's ability to cooperate in the feeding process. This is important whether the child is being fed by a carer or self-feeding. McEwan (1992) states that the goals of seating are to promote more functional movement, provide comfort, prevent skin breakdown and facilitate the child's involvement in a variety of environments. Pulmonary function (Nwaobi and Smith 1986) and digestion can be improved in children with cerebral palsy if appropriate support is provided (Zollars 1996).

While it is sometimes necessary to consider alternative positions for feeding, sitting is the primary position adopted. For some children suitable seating provides the stability and optimal posture required, while others may be more easily managed on their carer's lap. This can sometimes accommodate the child's physical needs most effectively and make it easier for the carer to feed the child. To decide on the optimum posture for feeding it is essential to complete a full examination of the child in relation to his or her sitting ability.

To resolve the child's seating needs is a complex problem-solving process which requires a specialist occupational therapist assessment.

Examination of oral-motor and pharyngeal mechanism

Crucial information regarding oral and pharyngeal function will be gathered during the general observation and the feeding observation. However, a more detailed assessment is usually required.

Oral motor control: the range and quality of oral motor movements at rest should be noted and a record made of any abnormal orofacial or tongue movements (e.g. dystonia). Mouth posture at rest, during speech and while eating and drinking should be noted as well as the frequency and extent of drooling. Providing the child is cognitively able, it is useful to ascertain if he or she can copy a range of movements and expressions and the accuracy, speed, range and quality of oral motor movements can be assessed. Many children with neurological deficits require extra time to be able to complete these tasks. If the child is unable to imitate oral movements then as full a range of movements as possible should be observed at rest and during feeding.

Oral motor function during feeding

Specific assessment of the oral motor mechanism is required to determine the child's ability to manage a range of different tastes and textures. Occasionally, clinicians may decide that the child is unsafe to feed orally and may defer any further oral assessment. However, it is possible to carry out an oral motor assessment in most children (providing they do not refuse food). There are, however, few standardised assessment tools that have demonstrated reliability or validity. Wolf and Glass (1998) review seven published feeding evaluations, comparing their scope and procedures. We recommend that any oral-motor assessment, whether a standardised protocol is adopted or not, should follow the principles outlined in the development of the Schedule for Oral Motor Assessment (SOMA, Reilly *et al.* 1995).

- Attention should be paid to achieving the best possible position prior to the assessment.
- Feeding utensils should be considered and in the case of children with neurological impairment, the most familiar utensil used in the first instance.
- The child's oral-motor skills should be challenged with a full range (where

possible) of tastes and textures, including liquids, purée, semi-solids, solids and chewy solids, such as biscuits or dried fruit.

• The manner in which the food and/or liquid is presented should be standardised so that a performance baseline can be established.

As well as difficulty managing liquids, many children with severe dysphagia are unable to manage foods that require chewing because of the lack of lateral tongue and jaw movements and inability to manipulate or transfer a bolus (for further details regarding specific oral-motor difficulties with textures readers are referred to Carroll and Reilly 1996). To summarise, the easiest and the safest textures for children with poor oral-motor skills are thick, cohesive purées.

Soft, easy-bite and dissolve foods, such as prawn crackers, Skips or Quavers, are often managed, even by children with moderate to severe dysphagia, providing they are placed carefully within the mouth. These textures provide sensory feedback when munched between the teeth, yet dissolve with saliva and do not require further chewing.

It is clear that for a thorough assessment of oral-motor function, a range of textures must be offered as ability can vary greatly. It is only through such detailed assessment that clinicians can decide on which textures the child is able to manage safely.

Pharyngeal function during feeding

An isolated clinical evaluation is of limited use in evaluating the swallowing mechanism in children with cerebral palsy. While gross swallowing problems may be detected, more subtle problems can be missed. For example, the clinical evaluation is only 50–66% accurate in determining the presence of aspiration (Splaingard *et al.* 1988) when compared to the gold standard, the modified barium swallow. This is partly because for many children aspiration is silent, that is, it is not accompanied by coughing and/or choking or any other signs that might alert carers to the fact that material is penetrating the airway.

Table 10.1 lists the main problems that occur in the pharyngeal stage of swallowing. Clinical signs and symptoms suggestive of swallowing dysfunction are outlined below:

• inability to manage secretions (drooling) and/or excessive oral and pharyngeal secretions
• audible upper airway sounds which can be described as 'wet' and 'bubbly' after swallowing. This may increase markedly during a feed
• multiple swallowing to clear a single bolus of food
• respiratory incoordination during feed

- apnoea during or after feeds
- marked inspiratory effort following a swallow
- auscultation of the swallow and associated breath sounds reveal deterioration in breath sounds and increase in noisy (wet and bubbly) airway sounds. (Auscultation implies listening to the swallow and breath sounds during feeding. A stethoscope is placed over the larynx and any change or deterioration in swallow or breath sounds noted)
- increasing congestion/wheeze during the feed
- eye tearing accompanied by gradual or sudden decrease in acceptance
- nasal regurgitation.

Coughing and choking are reflexive mechanisms that either prevent food and/ or liquid from entering the airway or expel food/liquid from the airway. The presence of coughing and choking during feeds may signify incoordination of the swallowing mechanism, particularly incoordination of respiration and swallowing. Coughing may also indicate that the child is attempting to protect his or her airway or that the child is trying to clear refluxed stomach contents from the airway or the pharynx.

The absence of coughing and choking is not, however, evidence of an adequate or safe swallow because aspiration may be silent. As a general rule, examination of the chest should be undertaken before, during and after feeding. Auscultation should include listening to the swallow and breath sounds associated with swallowing for any signs of deterioration in the clarity of breath sounds associated with feeding.

Laryngeal function

Laryngeal function cannot be assessed solely by clinical examination and observation. There is no doubt that diagnosis of any anatomical abnormality should be made by direct visualisation of the larynx. Clinical signs may alert the clinician to a swallowing problem as prolonged GOR resulting in aspiration can result in the vocal cords being 'bathed' in acid and affect vocal quality and result in a gruff or husky voice. Children who frequently aspirate or have excess secretions in or around the larynx often have 'wet-sounding' vocalisations. Vocal quality may also deteriorate during a feed and alert the clinician to the possibility of aspiration.

Observation of a feed

An assessment is incomplete unless a feed is observed. Watching a 'typical feed' with the parents/carers enables the clinician to verify much of the information reported (it should be checked that the observed feed is indeed representative). Ideally the observation should be undertaken in the home;

however, this is not always possible. An alternative is to ask the parents to video a meal time if this is possible. Parents are usually more than happy to bring food with them to the clinic appointment, particularly if they are asked in advance. The clinician is able to gain first-hand knowledge of the texture, amount and type of food the child is fed as well as how the child is positioned and managed during the meal.

The feeding observation alerts the clinician to how accurately and sensitively the parent/carer may be interpreting the child's signals during a meal and provides an indicator of how difficult the child is to feed. It may be a useful way of identifying symptoms which the parent has become accustomed to over the years. For example, in a recent interview, both parents of a severely disabled boy denied that he vomited and over the years had repeated this to many consultants who were querying if the boy may have had GOR. However, it became clear during the observation that the boy frequently regurgitated and vomited small amounts both throughout and after the meal. This was despite the parents' best efforts to keep him still and upright. When we asked if this was typical, both parents agreed 'he's always like this'; however, they did not recognise that the observed vomiting and regurgitation was abnormal or significant in their son since it had been happening for more than 10 years.

There are a number of ways in which parental reports and perceptions may not actually match the observational data. For example, in a study examining the feeding characteristics of a group of pre-school children with cerebral palsy, Reilly *et al.* (1996) found that the children's meals were in reality far shorter than mothers/carers perceived them to be. The more severe the child's dysphagia, the bigger the discrepancy; children with the more severe problems tended to have the shortest meal times. Clearly, how questions are asked is very important if clinicians are to elicit accurate information, but there is no substitute for the observation of a meal time in a child with dysphagia.

Further investigations

As a result of the clinical examination, some children with dysphagia will require further investigation. In the final section in this chapter we discuss the most common investigations undertaken in children with neurological problems and which children warrant further investigation.

Pointers to further investigation

Specific groups of children with neurological disease, namely those with four-limb involvement, are at greater risk of dysphagia. It is possible to identify clusters of signs and symptoms which, when combined with the type of cerebral palsy, identify a group likely to have severe dysphagia. This group is at risk of failing to thrive and of all the consequences of dysphagia described earlier in this chapter. The majority of these children will require further investigation.

Box 10.1: Signs and symptoms suggestive of a swallowing problem and aspiration that warrant further investigation

- Deterioration in respiratory status during feed/increased congestion
- Coughing and choking
- Noisy wet breath sounds
- History of wheeze and asthma
- History of chest infections/pneumonia
- Excessive pharyngeal secretions
- Structural chest abnormalities (e.g. Harrison's sulcus)
- Abnormalities of swallow and breath sounds on auscultation
- Evidence of premature over-spill in the oral stage
- Nasal regurgitation

Where a swallowing abnormality is suspected and aspiration may be a consequence, the existence of any single symptom may warrant further investigation, although in most cases there is more than likely to be a cluster of symptoms as outlined in Box 10.1. Similarly there are a number of signs and symptoms suggestive of GOR (Box 10.2) and these may be elicited during history taking or during the clinical examination.

Respiratory signs and symptoms may be indicative of aspiration, either as a result of a swallowing problem or as a result of GOR. It can be impossible to differentially diagnose between the two clinically without further investigation. Children presenting with any of the symptoms discussed should be considered for further investigations of their dysphagia.

Box 10.2: Signs and symptoms suggestive of gastro-oesophageal reflux

- Frequent spitting up, regurgitation, vomiting
- Discomfort, agitation and unexplained or abrupt mood changes during and after meals
- Sudden bouts of coughing/choking (may or may not be feed related)
- Excessive pharyngeal secretions/wet breath sounds
- Excessive, frequent swallowing
- Food refusal or fussy and particular about tastes and textures
- Abnormal posturing of the trunk, head, neck
- Poor, disrupted sleeping pattern
- Unexplained episodes or jerks that may resemble seizures
- History of wheeze and asthma
- History of chest infections/pneumonia
- Unexplained sleep apnoeas
- Frequent chest infections and pneumonia
- Increased congestion during feeds

Coordination of results

At the beginning of this chapter we highlighted the importance of the multidisciplinary team. It is vital that this approach extends throughout the assessment period and in discussion of the results. A problem-solving approach is necessary; results may not be clearcut and meaningful management strategies cannot be made in isolation. For example, a decision made solely on the basis of aspiration observed during a modified barium swallow could be very misleading; the barium swallow may not have been representative of the child's normal feeding pattern and there may be no other evidence or clinical signs and symptoms suggestive of aspiration in the child's history.

Summary

This chapter has discussed the main difficulties that prevent children with cerebral palsy from achieving an adequate intake of calories and the factors that sometimes make eating and drinking hazardous. It has highlighted the complexity of the problem, and the need for a multidisciplinary team and early diagnosis. Each stage of the feeding process in children with complex dysphagia must be carefully evaluated and then considered as part of the 'whole' picture. Chapter 11 discusses decision making and adoption of various management strategies. It is important to recognise, however, that these processes cannot occur until a detailed and thorough assessment has been undertaken.

References

Carr L, Reilly S and Cass H (1997) *A Paediatric Dysphagia Service: outcome in children with cerebral palsy.* American Academy of Cerebral Palsy and Developmental Disability, USA.

Carroll L and Reilly S (1996) The therapeutic approach to the child with feeding difficulties. II Management and treatment. In: L Rosenbloom and P Sullivan (eds) *Feeding the Disabled Child.* Clinics in Developmental Medicine. No. 140. MacKeith Press, London.

Claydon G (1996) Constipation in disabled children. In: L Rosenbloom and P Sullivan (eds) *Feeding the Disabled Child.* Clinics in Developmental Medicine. No. 140, pp 106–16. MacKeith Press, London.

Gisel EG (1992) Eating assessment and efficacy of oral-motor treatment in eating impaired children with cerebral palsy. *Cerebral Palsy Today.* **2**: 1–3.

Gisel EG and Patrick J (1988) Identification of children with cerebral palsy unable to maintain a normal nutritional state. *Lancet.* **1**: 283–6.

Hagberg B, Hagberg G, Olow I and von Wendt L (1996) The changing panorama of cerebral palsy in Sweden. VII. Prevalence and origin in the birth period 1987–1990. *Acta Paediatrica Scandinavica.* **85**: 954–60.

McEwan I (1992) Positioning for optimal AAC use: practical application of the research. ISAAC Biennial Conference, Philadelphia.

Nwaobi OM and Smith PD (1986) Effect of adaptive seating on pulmonary function of children with cerebral palsy. *Developmental Medicine and Child Neurology.* **28**: 351–4.

Patrick J and Gisel EJ (1990) Nutrition for the feeding impaired child. *Journal of Neurology and Rehabilitation.* **4**: 115–19.

Pelegrano JP, Nowysz S and Goesfered S (1994) Temporomandibular joint contractures in spastic quadriplegia: effect on oral-motor skills. *Developmental Medicine and Child Neurology.* **36**: 487–94.

Reilly S, Skuse D, Mathisen B and Wolke D (1995) The objective rating of oral-motor functions during feeding. *Dysphagia.* **10**: 177–91.

Reilly S, Skuse D and Poblete X (1996) Prevalence of feeding problems and oral-motor dysfunction in children with cerebral palsy: a community survey. *Journal of Pediatrics.* **129**(6): 877–82.

Rosenbloom L and Sullivan P (eds) (1996) *Feeding the Disabled Child.* Clinics in Developmental Medicine. No. 140. MacKeith Press, London.

Sandler ES, Roberts MW and Wojcicki AM (1974) Oral manifestations in a group of mentally retarded patients. *Journal of Dentistry for Children.* **41**: 207–11.

Sondheimer JM and Morris BA (1979) Gastro-eosophageal reflux among severely retarded children. *Journal of Pediatrics.* **94**: 710–14.

Splaingard ML, Hutchins B, Sulton HD and Chaudhuri G (1988) Aspiration in rehabilitation patients: videofluoroscopy vs bedside clinical assessment. *Archives of Physical Medicine and Rehabilitation.* **69**: 637–40.

Stallings VA, Charney EB, Davies JC and Cronk CE (1993) Nutrition related growth failure of children with quadriplegic cerebral palsy. *Developmental Medicine and Child Neurology.* **35**: 126–38.

Thommessan M, Heiberg A, Kase BF, Larsen S and Riis G (1991) Feeding problems, height and weight in different groups of disabled children. *Acta Paediatrica Scandinavica.* **80**: 527–33.

Wolf LS and Glass RP (1998) *Feeding and Swallowing Disorders in Infancy: assessment and management.* Psychological Corporation, Texas.

Zollars JA (1996) *Special Seating: an illustrated guide.* Ottobock Rehabilitation, Duderstadt/Eichsfeld.

Further reading

Bosma JF (1992) Pharyngeal swallow: basic mechanisms, development and impairments. *Advances in Otolaryngology Head and Neck Surgery.* **6**: 225–75.

Efthimiou J, Flemming J, Gomes C and Spiro SG (1988) The effect of supplementary oral nutrition in poorly nourished patients with chronic obstructive pulmonary disease. *American Review of Respiratory Disease.* **137**: 1075–82.

Groher ME (1994) Determination of the risks and benefits of oral feeding. *Dysphagia.* **9**: 233–5.

Logemann J (1983) *Manual for the videofluorographic study of swallowing.* Taylor & Francis, London.

Spender Q, Charney EB and Stallings VA (1989) Assessment of linear growth of children with cerebral palsy: use of alternative measures to height or length. *Developmental Medicine and Child Neurology.* **31**: 206–14.

CHAPTER 11

Approaches to managing feeding problems in children with neurological problems

Sheena Reilly, Alison Wisbeach and Lucinda Carr

Introduction

The management of dysphagia in children with neurological problems is complex. It should begin early in infancy as soon as problems become evident and continue throughout childhood and adolescence. Unfortunately, in many cases, children with dysphagia often come to the attention of the multi-disciplinary team late in childhood when crisis management may be necessary.

There are a variety of techniques and methods used for feeding children with neurological problems and dysphagia. Early intervention is advocated, not only for the child's health and well being but also for ease of management of the carers and family members. The management of feeding in the child with severe and complex neurological problems can raise difficult ethical issues for both health professionals and carers and these are touched on towards the end of this chapter, particularly in reference to the use of tube-feeding.

Prerequisites for managing dysphagia

There are four prerequisites for successful management. These are:

- a comprehensive assessment
- adopting a problem-solving approach
- assessment and management of dysphagia within the context of the child's other problems
- discussion and agreement of management regimes with parents/carers, other professionals and the child, if appropriate.

Each one is essential to the successful management of dysphagia in children with neurological problems. The multifactorial nature of dysphagia and thus the need for the skills and resources of a multidisciplinary team have already been highlighted in both this chapter and in Chapter 10, which focuses on assessment. For example, recommendations for modification of dietary intake in young children with cerebral palsy may be made by a dietician or a speech and language therapist. The dietician may recommend increased fibre and roughage or particular types of food. The speech and language therapist knows the child will not be able to manage particular textures because of the degree of oral and pharyngeal dysphagia. However, together the dietician and speech and language therapist can plan a dietary regime that is both appropriate in terms of nutritional intake and safe in regard to the texture the child can manage. A common recommendation for many children with cerebral palsy is to increase liquid intake; however, liquids are the most difficult texture to manage for those with oral and/or pharyngeal dysphagia. Any increase therefore may be detrimental to the child's pulmonary status because the child may be at risk of aspiration. The speech therapist together with the dietician may therefore recommend that liquids are increased but only if they are thickened. Clearly management of such issues requires discussion and decision making among the team.

Comprehensive assessment

A comprehensive assessment is crucial to establish a baseline of abilities and difficulties against which change can be measured and as a basis on which to develop treatment regimes. Both the clinical examination and the diagnostic work-up should include assessment of all potential causes of dysphagia in the child with cerebral palsy. As previously highlighted, gastro-oesophageal reflux (GOR) occurs commonly in cerebral palsy and should therefore always be excluded in the child with four-limb involvement. Failure to detect significant reflux in a child recommended for gastrostomy can result in frequent vomiting and regurgitation postoperatively as a result of the increased volume of feed. Consequently the child may experience more frequent chest infections and/or respiratory problems and ongoing pain, discomfort and anxiety.

Adopting a problem-solving approach

Differential diagnosis is rarely straightforward in the child with multiple and complex difficulties. It is often necessary to problem solve as part of the management process because the aetiology of the presenting symptomatology may not always be clear. A dilemma for paediatricians and neurologists may present in the child with epilepsy, suspected GOR and dystonic spasms. These episodes can appear very similar in the child with complex and multiple disabilities. Sudden, jerky movements may be the result of seizure activity, an episode of GOR or a spasm. Careful evaluation and where possible simultaneous monitoring (e.g. electroencephalogram (EEG) and pH monitoring) may be necessary to fully understand the presenting problem.

Management within the context of the child's other multiple and complex problems

Sometimes it is necessary to set priorities for management. While some interventions may be independent, others are closely interlinked and may be dependent on the outcome of each other.

In the child with complex and multiple needs there may be competing surgical needs. For example, a tonsillectomy and adenoidectomy may have been recommended as well as surgery for hips and spine. In addition, the child may also require a gastrostomy. Clearly each recommendation must be carefully evaluated and listed in order of priority. A tonsillectomy and adenoidectomy may need to be performed to ensure a patent airway. A gastrostomy may be a priority because of the child's nutritional needs and orthopaedic surgery may therefore be postponed until the child is in a better nutritional state.

Appropriate seating is almost always a priority to ensure that the child can feed safely and adequately. Oral-motor control and postural control are very closely related. Therefore oral-motor therapy may not be fully instigated until the child's seating needs and equipment have been provided as successful oral-motor therapy is almost completely dependent on the child's stable and safe positioning.

Discuss and agree regimes with parents/carers and the child if appropriate

Unless care plans are discussed openly and fully with parents and professional colleagues and their views considered, treatments are likely to fail. There are limited benefits to carrying out interventions solely in the school or treatment centre environments; even children in full-time education spend less than a third of their day at school. This may of course be necessary in some cases but clinicians should be aware of the limitations of this approach. Ideally parents need to be in full agreement with the proposed management, understand the rationale behind it and be able to integrate it into home life. The provision of equipment, such as specialised seating, can be costly. If parents are not fully included in the decision-making process about equipment they may feel it has been imposed on them and they are less likely to use it. This was clearly illustrated in a pilot study of feeding patterns in children with cerebral palsy (Reilly and Skuse 1992). Only half of the children observed at meal times were actually fed in the seating provided or prescribed by occupational therapists and physiotherapists. As a result many of the children were very poorly positioned during meal times. Some mothers described the equipment as a nuisance and cumbersome to use, others found it impractical or uncomfortable to use. In just over a quarter of families the equipment was not used but was stored in a cupboard or another part of the house. If we are to be successful, parents do need to be partners in deciding on methods of treatment and choosing equipment. An investment is therefore required from all health professionals working with the family to ensure that this is possible. This may require extra time so that families are clear about the priorities for their child and the rationale for deciding on management regimes.

Decision making

One of the first and often most crucial decisions about feeding dysphagic children is whether the child can be fed orally. Both the safety and adequacy of continued oral feeding must be taken into account as well as current dietary management. For children unable to achieve an adequate intake via oral means, non-oral methods of feeding might be considered to supplement nutrition taken orally. This may include nasogastric tube-feeds (used for short-term feeding supplementation) or gastrostomy tube-feeding (used for long-term feeding problems). Decisions regarding the continuation of oral feeding or alternative methods to be used can only be made after a thorough assessment. Failure to do so can result in poor outcome for the child and family. Figure 11.1 outlines the problem-solving approach developed and adopted by the paediatric dysphagia clinic at Great Ormond Street Children's Hospital. Clearly the questions posed can only be answered after a comprehensive assessment has been performed, as outlined in Chapter 10.

Specific management strategies

Positioning and seating

For the child to have the best opportunity to participate in the feeding process, appropriate positioning is essential. To identify the most suitable seating for the child it is necessary to assess his or her physical status and functional

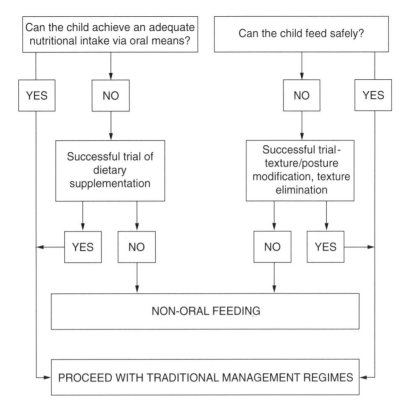

Figure 11.1: Decision making: considering the safety and adequacy of oral feeding in children with dysphagia.

abilities. This will include joint mobility, particularly of the hips, knees and ankles, shoulder girdle and spine, and skin condition. Functional assessment will include the child's saving and balance reactions, sitting ability, head control and hand use. For children with deformities it is important to identify whether or not these are fixed or mobile, and the plans for their management within the context of the child's overall postural management.

To gain sufficient information to decide on the most appropriate seat it may be necessary for the child to be seen by a team of professionals who focus on spinal and postural management, since the options for treatment are complex and may include:

- spinal surgery/hip surgery
- spinal bracing
- dynamic Lycra splinting
- special seating

- pressure relief cushioning
- 24-hour postural management.

It is also essential to take into account the physical measurements of the child since this will help in identifying the correct seat size.

The range of potential seating solutions is ever-changing, with new systems being introduced to the market all the time. The principles on which these seats are designed fall broadly into three categories:

- standard seating
- adaptive seating
- moulded seat.

Standard seating

These are conventional seats with support offered only from the seat and backrest. A child would need to have good independent sitting abilities and it would be unlikely that children with complex dysphagia would be sufficiently skilled to use these.

Adaptive seating

These systems are flexible. They comprise individual postural supports within a seat system enabling the individual seat to be customised by selecting size, shape and placement of support.

Moulded seating

These are intimate contour seats for maximum support and are suitable for the most involved movement disorders.

Based on the child's physical and functional needs and dimension then the type of seating system can be identified. To help select the seat system from within the category, other considerations must be taken into account. These will include the following social and environmental considerations:

- acceptability by the child and carers
- reliability
- durability
- ease of use
- space within the home
- manoeuvrability
- access
- steps or stairs

- door widths
- transportability in the family, at school and vehicle access
- storage facilities
- heights of tables/chairs for interaction.

Although some children are provided with a chair purely for feeding, it is more usual for the chair to be used for school and leisure activities as well. Once the seating system has been provided and is agreed to be suitable, the child will need to be gradually introduced to the system to give both the child and carers time to accommodate. During this time observations should be made of the effect stimulation/activity has on the child's sitting. It may be necessary to make adjustments during this period. Once the child appears comfortable and relaxed in his or her chair then oral feeding may be introduced. It is important to review the seat regularly to ensure that it continues to meet the child's needs.

Management of oral-sensorimotor problems

Oral-sensorimotor treatment aims to improve oral-motor control of food and liquid thereby focusing on areas such as tongue lateralisation, lip and jaw control, and vigour of chewing. Techniques vary widely but have included: physical/manual manipulation of the tongue, lips and jaw in an attempt to encourage chewing and or munching, specific exercises designed to encourage and practise lip-rounding; particular activities to encourage a wider range of tongue movements, such as placing tastes at the outer lip margins; and encouraging the child to lick the substance or placing food directly on to the teeth in attempt to encourage chewing. Clinicians and researchers may ask why we are discussing oral-sensorimotor treatment since almost no evidence exists to prove its efficacy. One of the most widely quoted and well-known studies (Ottenbacher *et al.* 1983) showed no change in oral-motor function or weight gain after a nine-week intensive sensorimotor training period. Erika Gisel (1996) suggested possible explanations for the failure to demonstrate change. First, many studies included children with a range of oral-motor impairments (from mild to severe) and did not focus on a particular group. Second, the specific oral-sensorimotor techniques used in many of the studies varied considerably. Third, different outcomes measures were used to judge success.

Gisel (1996) designed a study to address these problems. She chose a group of children with cerebral palsy defined as having moderate eating impairment to test the efficacy of specific and clearly defined oral-sensorimotor treatment. The findings of her study are significant. She compared children who had received oral-sensorimotor treatment with those who did not. Her findings are summarised below.

- There was no significant decrease in the mean meal-time duration of the treatment groups.
- Some children were able to advance from soft, mashed textures to more solid textures during the treatment period.
- There was no catch-up growth during the treatment period, although the children maintained their weight.

Gisel (1996) argued that longer treatment periods may result in significant change given the trends demonstrated in the study. Although she has shown that there are some benefits to oral-sensorimotor therapy, it is important to consider the cost and benefits carefully. For example, what is the cost of encouraging a more highly textured diet that results in longer meal times for the child with cerebral palsy who is underweight? Common sense tells us that it takes longer to eat foods that require vigorous chewing and may fatigue some children. The increased effort and extra time taken (for both the child and carer) to eat more solid foods *must* be balanced against the child's nutritional requirements, which remain paramount.

Many different oral-sensorimotor techniques have been developed over the years and some of those used for children with neurological impairment are illustrated in Table 11.1. Applying the appropriate management strategy is wholly dependent on understanding the problem, which is only possible after a comprehensive assessment. Oral motor treatment strategies must be applied in conjunction with managing posture and position for eating and drinking. For example, traditional methods for managing poor lip closure include the provision of jaw support while firmly helping to keep the lips closed using the therapist's fingers. Not surprisingly the technique was often not successful because the therapist was treating only the most visible component of the problem. Providing manual lip closure will be unsuccessful in the child with a malocclusion (because of the structural abnormality). In the child with postural instability, correction may allow the child to develop jaw stability without the need for manual assistance.

There are several reasons why children with cerebral palsy may have difficulty retaining food and/or liquid in the mouth. The child's posture may be such that gravity contributes to liquid/food loss. Structural abnormalities, such as malocclusions or fixed contractures of the jaw, may make closure impossible or very difficult. They may not be able to collect up the liquid/food placed in the mouth. Limited tongue movements (for example extension and retraction movements only) might result in some of the liquid/food being accidentally expelled. The problem may be texture specific; that is, there may be greater loss with liquids than with solids. The inability to transport the

Table 11.1: The management of common oral motor problems in children with dysphagia

Stage	Problem	Management strategy
Oral	Poor absent bolus formation	Modify texture – deliver a cohesive bolus that does not spread throughout the oral cavity
	Poor/absent transportation of bolus	Place bolus carefully within the oral cavity to facilitate swallow initiation*
	Poor/absent manipulation of bolus	Dependent on texture therefore modify texture as necessary and consider bolus placement
	Poor/absent tongue lateralisation/ elevation, etc.	Place food directly on to molars or gum margins Avoid food which requires munching and/or chewing if child is not able to manage safely

	Poor/absent ability to retain food/ liquid bolus within oral cavity	Consider total body position, in particular head and neck position. Modify seating if necessary, to avoid loss due to gravity
		    Modify texture – thicker textures may result in reduced loss as compared to liquids
		    Consider bolus placement

	Poor/absent lip closure	Modify position – ensure child has postural stability Assist with manual lip closure
	Poor/absent jaw closure	Modify position – ensure child has postural stability Provide jaw support
	Lumps swallowed whole	Place food directly on to molars Avoid
	Lumps manipulated but not masticated	Avoid
	Lumps remain stationary on the tongue	Avoid Try placing food on to molars
	Premature overspill into pharynx	Modify texture – thicken to slow down passage of bolus Alter method of delivery to slow down pace

* This can only be achieved if there is sufficient mouth opening and the child is tolerant of posterior bolus placement.

bolus through the oral cavity may result in the food/liquid remaining on the front of the tongue until it is expelled or falls out.

These examples illustrate that there can be many reasons underlying the presenting oral-motor problem. It is therefore necessary to manage such problems not only from a multidisciplinary perspective but also to be aware that there may be multiple factors contributing to the presenting problem.

Management of pharyngeal dysphagia

In 95% of the referred sample of children with cerebral palsy studied by Mirrett *et al.* (1994) both the oral and pharyngeal stages were found to be abnormal. Although oral- and pharyngeal-stage problems can occur independently of each other, severe oral-stage problems can lead to pharyngeal problems. For example, the inability to control a bolus in the oral stage can result in premature overspill into the pharynx and result in aspiration prior to the swallow being triggered. If the oral stage can be controlled (for example by slowing down the bolus and improving bolus formation) there may be no aspiration and no evidence of pharyngeal dysphagia. It is important therefore to carefully evaluate each stage to ascertain if both stages are affected and if so, to what extent.

Given that the consequences of pharyngeal-stage dysphagia can affect morbidity and mortality significantly, by definition, the strategies employed are more aggressive and it is often necessary to consider non-oral methods of feeding sooner rather than later. The decision-making process is outlined in Figure 11.1, and in Table 11.2 the most common pharyngeal-stage problems are shown along with appropriate management strategies.

Management of oesophageal-stage problems

Medical management

The presence of GOR and/or constipation first requires consultation with a paediatrician and/or gastroenterologist. A phased therapeutic approach to the management of GOR is recommended by Vanenplas *et al.* (1993) and Lloyd and Pierro (1996). Three phases are outlined: in phase 1, attention is given to position, dietary advice and thickening agents. Traditionally, thickening feeds and the maintenance of an upright position after feeds were encouraged; however, these are no longer thought to be effective in children with neurological disorder. In addition, antacids, such as Gaviscon to neutralise the gastric acid and sucralfate to protect the mucosa, may be added.

In phase 2, prokinetic agents, such as cisapride, which increase the tone of the lower oesophageal sphincter and enhance gastric emptying may be added. Acid production may be further reduced by both H2 receptor blockers and more powerful proton pump inhibitors if there are persistent oesophageal symptoms. The outcome for medical management of GOR in children with neurological problems is known to be less effective than in neurologically normal children. Some children fail to respond to medical management of GOR as may be illustrated by the persistence or worsening of symptoms. Surgical management may therefore need consideration and will be discussed later in this chapter.

Table 11.2: The management of pharyngeal dysphagia in children with cerebral palsy

Stage	Problem	Management strategy
Pharyngeal	Aspiration/penetration before swallow	Improve bolus formation in the oral stage, by modifying texture, pacing delivery and altering bolus size Alter head position to change calibre of airway. Chin tuck may be useful

	Aspiration/penetration during swallow	Alter head position to change calibre of airway. Chin tuck may be useful
		  Change utensil – an angled bottle is sometimes useful
		  Supraglottic swallow might be useful for children who are cognitively able

	Aspiration/penetration after swallow	Dry swallow to clear pharyngeal residue
		  Liquids may be given to clear residue if safe
		  Modify consistency – feed foods that cause least amount of residue and pooling
		  Encourage non-nutritive sucking after swallow
		  Palatal training devices reported to be useful

	Absent swallow reflex	Do not feed orally
	Delayed swallow reflex	Improve bolus formation in the oral stage, by modifying texture, pacing delivery and altering bolus size Thermal stimulation is useful in some situations
	Pooling of food/liquid in valleculae or pyriform sinus	Alter head position to decrease size of valleculae thus reducing likelihood of pooling – use with caution
	Reduced pharyngeal peristalsis	Modify texture

	Nasal regurgitation	Alter head position
		  Modify texture – avoid those which cause significant regurgitation
		  Palatal training device

	Delayed/absent cricopharyngeal relaxation	Surgical – cricopharyngeal myotomy
		  Dilation of the cricopharyngeus
		  Botulinum toxin injections

	Poorly coordinated ventilatory cycle and swallowing	Discourage post-swallow inspiration Supraglottic swallow

Nutritional intervention

Nutritional management of the severely disabled child has in the past been neglected. This has occurred largely because of a number of misconceptions regarding the growth of children with neurological involvement. For many years growth failure was accepted as an inevitable and irremediable consequence of cerebral palsy. It is only relatively recently that it has been shown that undernutrition is often a major cause of this growth failure (due in part to the severe oral and pharyngeal dysphagia which restricts the child's caloric intake). Furthermore, the malnutrition is correctable.

Nutritional therapy should be part of the child's comprehensive care and rehabilitation. It aims not only to improve weight and linear growth but to improve physiological and functional capacity. Very little is known about the specific nutrient requirements of children with developmental disabilities or those with different types of motor disorders. For example, a child with excessive involuntary movements (e.g. athetosis) is thought to have increased energy needs, whereas some immobile children with four-limb involvement may have much lower energy requirements.

Caloric requirements are usually estimated from Recommended Daily Allowances (RDAs). However, RDAs assume normal levels of activity and are therefore not appropriate for children with complex and multiple disabilities. There are a variety of methods used to calculate energy requirements in the child with complex and multiple disabilities. Some clinicians recommend that energy requirements be based on the RDA for their height, age or their weight at the 25th percentile weight for height. Others recommend determining basal metabolic rates which are corrected for activity levels, such as the World Health Organisation formulae which allow for more individualised prediction based on gender, age and body weight as well as accounting for activity levels. Two further methods for the estimation of calorie requirements have been published by Culley and Middleton (1969) and Krick *et al.* (1992). The first takes into account the child's level of motor function, whereas Krick and colleagues (1992) developed a factorial approach based on estimating resting energy expenditure needs, muscle tone alterations, normal growth needs and catch-up growth or nutritional repletion in malnourished children.

It is crucial that a paediatric dietician experienced in the management of children with multiple and complex needs be part of the team to evaluate and establish nutritional plans for each child. Monitoring these plans is of vital importance to ensure that children reach the expected growth targets. However, in the case of some children, particularly those who are gastrostomy fed, it may be necessary to ensure that they do not exceed weight targets.

Utensils

Part of managing dysphagia, particularly the oral phase, involves modifying the manner in which food and/or liquid is delivered and placed in the mouth. This often means experimenting with different types of cup and spoon. As a general rule non-metallic utensils are advised for the child's comfort and safety. Spoons and cups should be non-breakable as some children with cerebral palsy may bite on the spoon or glass, which can be dangerous. In addition, cold metallic spoons can be uncomfortable and cause pain if not placed carefully, coming in contact with sensitive teeth or sore mouths. The sudden, uncontrolled movements of some children mean that teeth and gums can contact painfully with metallic utensils despite the carer's best efforts.

For the young child with cerebral palsy who is capable of sucking from a bottle there is a range of teats available, including vented teats that help prevent air-swallowing. These are recommended. Soft, squeeze bottles, such as the Mead Johnson (used for babies with cleft lip and palate), may also help when the suck is weak. Care needs to be taken not to flood the baby's mouth and pharynx. However, for many babies with cerebral palsy the suck is so weak that this becomes an inefficient method of feeding when the energy and time spent on feeding are measured against the effort. For this reason, early cup-feeding is often appropriate. Small, plastic, medicine cups or soft, flexible cups are often very useful. Alternatively, soft trainer spouts are now available, and providing the baby can manage the flow of liquid they can be very successful. The liquid may also be thickened if necessary to slow the flow.

There is a wide range of spoons available, in various shapes, bowl depths, sizes and material. The type chosen depends largely on the individual child. Small teaspoons coated with a soft plastic are often suitable for the young child taking his or her first solids. A variety of weaning spoons, some with flat bowls and others with deep bowls, is available. They may be either long- or short-handled. Spoons made of bone are also available and suit the requirements of certain children, although they are costly and can be hard to find. Bowl size should be determined by the size of the child's mouth. For children aversive to spoons or those taking very small tastes of food, small plastic spatulas can be used.

Self-feeding

For some children with cerebral palsy independence in self-feeding is not possible. Both Reilly *et al.* (1996) and Thomas *et al.* (1989) found that a high proportion of individuals with cerebral palsy (60% and 56% respectively) had major difficulties in self-feeding. Decisions to introduce self-feeding must be carefully assessed in conjunction with assessment of joint mobility, balance and type of seating. While encouraging independence at meal times is desirable, it must be carefully balanced against an individual's nutritional needs and the time taken to feed. For some children the effort to maintain stability and initiate hand-to-mouth actions can cause a decrease in oral-motor control and result in loss of food and/or liquid.

Some children are determined to self-feed. To achieve maximum independence, careful consideration should be given to their posture and position. The relationship of the table and/or tray to the child is vital. It must be of the correct height and position; this is especially important if the child is to stabilise or fix one arm on the tray while feeding with the other. Reach, grasp and hand-to-mouth ability require careful evaluation, and modification of equipment and position may be necessary to accommodate any difficulties. The pace of feeding and delivery of food often change when a child begins to self-feed and it may be necessary to provide verbal prompts to encourage the child to take 1–2 mouthfuls before pausing. Similarly, head position may alter during self-feeding with the result that the child extends his or her head further back as the spoon approaches, resulting in unsafe practices. All these aspects of self-feeding require monitoring if the child is going to be able to feed safely and take in an adequate amount. It may of course be necessary to continue a combination of dependent and independent feeding and it is sometimes helpful to target less stressful times, such as snack periods, to encourage self-feeding.

There are a number of aids for self-feeding. These include aids that reduce the physical demands necessary to self-feed, such as the Neat-a-eater (Neater Solutions Ltd, Michaelis Engineering Ltd, 13 Spencer Road, Buxton, Derbyshire) and robotic devices, which may enable more dependent children capable of using switches to feed themselves. However, these are not without drawbacks. The devices tend to be bulky and therefore not readily transportable (some are too bulky to be moved) and are not able to manage a wide range of food sizes and textures.

Communication/behaviour/interaction

There are many reasons why difficulty communicating complicates the feeding problems in children with cerebral palsy. Owing to severely delayed and/or disordered speech development, many children are unable to request food or drink, make their preferences known, tell if food is offered too fast or too slow, or explain how the process feels. Imagine yourself unable to let your feeder know that you loathe spinach, yet you find it is on the menu every lunch time! Some children may have a means of communicating either verbally or non-verbally (e.g. eye-pointing, gestures), but their attempts may not be easily interpreted. Awareness and sensitivity to the child's method of communication is therefore important. This should include being aware of any non-verbal messages such as change in the child's facial expression, body posture and mood. Understanding and attending to communicative behaviours is time-consuming and demanding for the feeder, who must remember to give the child choices and create opportunities for communication. When not given some means of communication it is not surprising that children with cerebral palsy can develop difficult behaviour at meal times.

The child with cerebral palsy may also develop interactional and/or behaviour problems associated with eating and drinking. However, careful assessment should always aim to eliminate the possibility of any underlying organic deficit for food refusal or other aversive behaviours evident at meal times. Feeding children with dysphagia can be stressful for their parents and carers and is often not a pleasant experience. The children may cough and choke excessively, lose a large proportion of each mouthful, and regurgitate and vomit feeds. In many cases mothers remain solely responsible for feeding their child, adding to the already considerable burden of care. The provision of respite care or support for relief from feeding can be helpful.

Parents whose child has been diagnosed as having cerebral palsy may have a sense of loss akin to bereavement. There may be ongoing, unresolved grief for the 'normal' child they have lost and anger, particularly if the events surrounding the birth were distressing. In some circumstances parents may not recognise that their child has severe difficulties feeding or may deny that these problems exist. Depression is known to affect a mother's ability to communicate with her child and can therefore influence how well she is able to feed her child (Reilly and Skuse 1992). Clinicians need to be aware of potential problems and be prepared to offer support and arrange counselling where necessary.

Non-oral feeding

The safety of oral feeding is essential. It is often the most pressing issue yet also the most difficult to evaluate and manage in children with dysphagia. The results of the clinical examination, dietetics evaluation, videofluoroscopy and chest X-ray contribute to the decision-making process as outlined in Figure 11.1.

In children with cerebral palsy it is sometimes necessary to consider non-oral methods of feeding. Factors which may contribute to the decision-making process are listed in Box 11.1.

Box 11.1: Reasons for considering non-oral feeding in children with cerebral palsy

- The child is unable to consume adequate calories orally to meet energy requirements
- There is evidence of ongoing aspiration during oral feeding
- Oral feeding is stressful for either the carer or the child or both
- Meal times are protracted leaving limited time for other daily activities
- Oral supplementation of the diet has failed
- Chronic food refusal or aversive behaviour has developed
- Oral intake is erratic
- Child needs safe route for regular medication (e.g. anti-convulsants)

Nasogastric verses gastrostomy feeding

Nasogastric tubes enter the gastrointestinal tract via the nose. Recent developments have resulted in the availability of a much larger range of tubes, including fine-bore silk tubes which are relatively easy to insert and can be left *in situ* for longer periods. Nasogastric feeding is often the first choice if enteral feeding is required because it is less invasive and viewed as a temporary measure. Either continuous or bolus feeds may be given and the tube can be used to top up or supplement oral intake.

Disadvantages include the fact that the tube is highly visible and therefore unaesthetic. Continued use may cause nasopharyngeal discomfort and the tube may block or become dislodged. The presence of the tube is also said to promote GOR by the very fact that larger volume feeds are now being introduced into the stomach. In children with severe GOR the tube may be constantly dislodged because of frequent vomiting, regurgitation and retching. Over time, toleration of the tube decreases in some children to the extent that they may constantly pull the tube out, either deliberately or randomly with extraneous movements. Parents need to be proficient in placing the tubes.

Most clinicians would agree that nasogastric tubes should be used for short-term feeding and some would advocate it should not be used to manage dysphagia in children with cerebral palsy for longer than 12 weeks. The need for prolonged tube-feeding is indicative of a long-term problem requiring a long-term solution. For this reason gastrostomy feeding is recommended for children who require ongoing supplementary feeding.

Gastrostomy tubes may be placed surgically or by a percutaneous technique with endoscopic guidance. Further details of the exact procedures are given in Lloyd and Pierro (1996). The indications for gastrostomy insertion are basically the same as those already highlighted for tube-feeding, although some additional reasons exist, as discussed in Chapter 2.

Surgical management of gastro-oesophageal reflux

Surgical management of GOR is a major undertaking and not without potential complications in the child with multiple and complex disabilities. There are a number of different surgical procedures. Those most commonly recommended for children with neurological problems include the Nissen's fundoplication and the Thal fundoplication. Descriptions of both procedures may be found in Lloyd and Pierro (1996). Both involve wrapping the fundus of the stomach around the distal oesophagus. Chapter 2 summarises surgical interventions, as well as their complications.

Protocols for managing unsafe oral feeding

The management of aspiration challenges all clinicians working with dysphagic children and their families. It is important to remember that aspiration is a symptom of dysphagia and not a condition in itself. There is much that we do not understand about managing children who aspirate. However, there is no doubt that it should never be managed in isolation. The whole child must be considered in decision making and management strategies implemented with the knowledge and agreement of the whole team. Wolf and Glass (1992) established four treatment strategies for infants and children who aspirate. In the Paediatric Dysphagia Clinic we have adapted and modified them for use with children who have complex and multiple disabilities (*see* Figure 11.2). They help to form the basis for decision making regarding oral feeding and provide a rationale for the approach adopted for the child's parents, carers and other professionals.

Conclusion

In 1989 Martin Bax, a distinguished paediatrician, wrote an editorial entitled 'Feeding is important'. He asked why 'feeding', in particular how to get food into young children, had received such scant attention in the paediatric medical literature. He suggested that this apparent neglect might be attributed to the fact that the topic was adequately covered in general childcare books and was therefore not seen as a 'respectable' one worthy of attention in paediatric textbooks. Almost 10 years later professional attitudes to feeding the disabled child have changed significantly. Clinicians are now aware of the importance

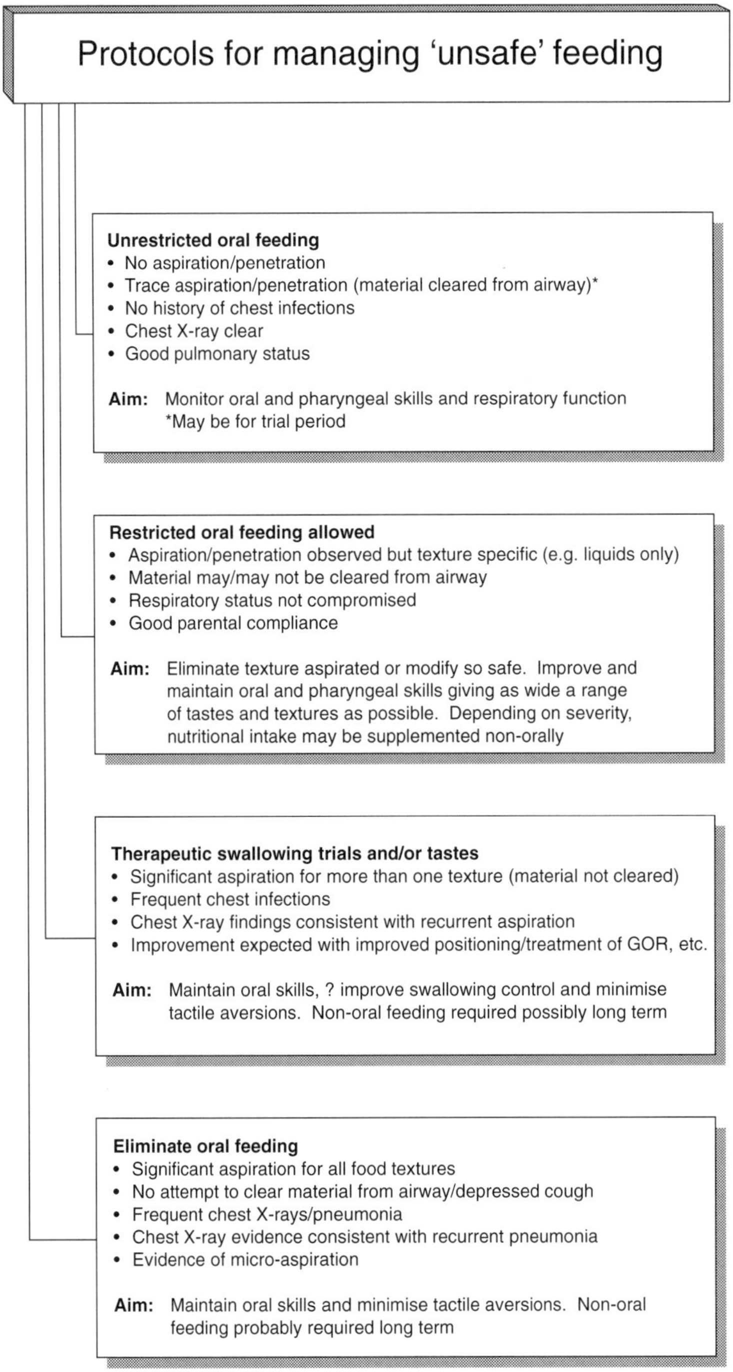

Protocols for managing 'unsafe' feeding

Unrestricted oral feeding
- No aspiration/penetration
- Trace aspiration/penetration (material cleared from airway)*
- No history of chest infections
- Chest X-ray clear
- Good pulmonary status

Aim: Monitor oral and pharyngeal skills and respiratory function
*May be for trial period

Restricted oral feeding allowed
- Aspiration/penetration observed but texture specific (e.g. liquids only)
- Material may/may not be cleared from airway
- Respiratory status not compromised
- Good parental compliance

Aim: Eliminate texture aspirated or modify so safe. Improve and maintain oral and pharyngeal skills giving as wide a range of tastes and textures as possible. Depending on severity, nutritional intake may be supplemented non-orally

Therapeutic swallowing trials and/or tastes
- Significant aspiration for more than one texture (material not cleared)
- Frequent chest infections
- Chest X-ray findings consistent with recurrent aspiration
- Improvement expected with improved positioning/treatment of GOR, etc.

Aim: Maintain oral skills, ? improve swallowing control and minimise tactile aversions. Non-oral feeding required possibly long term

Eliminate oral feeding
- Significant aspiration for all food textures
- No attempt to clear material from airway/depressed cough
- Frequent chest X-rays/pneumonia
- Chest X-ray evidence consistent with recurrent pneumonia
- Evidence of micro-aspiration

Aim: Maintain oral skills and minimise tactile aversions. Non-oral feeding probably required long term

Figure 11.2: Protocols for managing 'unsafe' feeding.

of ensuring that children with cerebral palsy are adequately nourished. This has resulted in the adoption of a variety of different management strategies, including the increasing use of surgical placement of feeding tubes.

However, these changes have also raised ethical dilemmas for clinicians regarding nutritional intervention in children with severe cerebral palsy. The use of gastrostomy feeding in this population seems to have become a particularly contentious issue for both professionals and parents. In discussing the ethics and implications of treatment programmes for disabled children with feeding problems, Rosenbloom and Sullivan (1996) state that:

> the provision of appropriate nutrition has to be set within the context of their overall needs, their prognosis and the perceptions and wishes of their parents and other carers.

Clearly there is a range of complex ethical issues for parents, carers and the professionals involved with the child's care and it is beyond the scope of this chapter to expand further. It is, however, vital that clinicians working with children who have cerebral palsy are familiar with the different treatment methods and with the complex management issues that may arise.

References

Bax MCO (1989) Eating is important (editorial). *Developmental Medicine and Child Neurology.* **31**: 285–6.

Culley WJ and Middleton TO (1969) Caloric requirements of mentally retarded children with and without motor dysfunction. *Journal of Pediatrics.* **75**: 380–4.

Gisel EG (1996) Effect of sensorimotor treatment on measures of growth and efficiency of eating in the moderately eating-impaired child with cerebral palsy. *Dysphagia.* **11**: 59–71.

Krick J, Murphy PE, Markham JFB and Shapiro BK (1992) A proposed formula for calculating energy needs of children with cerebral palsy. *Developmental Medicine and Child Neurology.* **34**: 481–7.

Lloyd DA and Pierro A (1996). The therapeutic approach to the child with feeding difficulty: III Enteral feeding. In: L Rosenbloom and P Sullivan (eds) *Feeding the Disabled Child.* Clinics in Developmental Medicine. No. 140, pp 132–50. MacKeith Press, London.

Mirrett PL, Riski JE, Glascott MA and Johnson V (1994) Videofluoroscopic assessment of dysphagia in children with severe spastic cerebral palsy. *Dysphagia.* **9**: 174–9.

Ottenbacher K, Bundy A and Short MA (1983) The development and treatment of oral-motor dysfunction: a review of clinical research. *Physical and Occupational Therapy in Pediatrics.* **3**: 147–60.

Reilly S and Skuse D (1992) Characteristics and management of feeding problems in young children with cerebral palsy. *Developmental Medicine and Child Neurology.* **34**: 379–88.

Reilly S, Skuse D and Poblete X (1996) Prevalence of feeding problems and oral motor dysfunction in children with cerebral palsy: a community survey. *Journal of Pediatrics.* **129**(6): 877–82.

Rosenbloom L and Sullivan P (eds) (1996) *Feeding the Disabled Child.* Clinics in Developmental Medicine. No. 140. MacKeith Press, London.

Thomas AP, Bax MCO and Smyth D (1989) *The health and social needs of young adults with physical disabilities.* Clinics in Developmental Medicine. No. 106. MacKeith Press, London.

Vanenplas Y, Ashkenazi A, Bellie D, Boige N, Bouquet J, Cadranel S, Cezard JP, Cuccharia S and Dupont C (1993) A proposition for the diagnosis and treatment of gastro-oesophageal reflux disease in children: a report from a working group on gastro-oesophageal reflux disease. *European Journal of Pediatrics.* **152**: 704–11.

Wolf LS and Glass RP (1992) *Feeding and Swallowing Disorders in Infancy: assessment and management.* Therapy Skill Builders, Tucson, Arizona.

CHAPTER 12

Interventions with children who are tube-fed

Mandy Bryon

Introduction

Feeding and eating difficulties in young children are common, with reports that they occur in over 20% of normal infants (Lindberg *et al.* 1991; Reau *et al.* 1996). They are so common that we may find ourselves differentiating between 'normal feeding difficulties' and 'severe feeding difficulties'. Children who are tube-fed would appear to be at the severe end of the spectrum. However, infants and young children may require all or some of their nutrition delivered artificially via a tube for one basic reason: they are unable to consume sufficient calories for adequate growth orally. The reasons for this vary widely, but the point is that tube-feeding is a simple solution to a potentially serious problem. It is, therefore, likely to be an increasingly common phenomenon seen in local clinics and not just major paediatric centres.

Tube-feeding is the delivery of a liquid nutritional formula to the infant or child by a tube. The place of entry of the tube varies according to the physical condition of the child and the length of time tube-feeding is planned. Types of tube-feeding are: nasogastric tube-feeding, where a tube is passed through the nose and into the stomach; nasojejunum tube-feeding, where a tube is passed through the nose into some other part of the gut, for example, the jejunum; gastrostomy feeding where a tube is passed, surgically, into the stomach with the end protruding from the surface of the body; and total parenteral nutrition (TPN), where a tube is passed directly into the bloodstream. The decision to feed a child via a tube is a medical decision and such children often have a physical condition which makes oral feeding or absorption of nutrition deficient or impossible.

Tube-feeding can be prescribed in conjunction with a wide range of paediatric organic conditions (Linscheid *et al.* 1995). Diseases such as severe chronic renal failure invariably require some form of tube-feeding (Strologo *et al.* 1997). Some, relatively common, gastroenterological conditions may require temporary tube-feeding: for example gastroenteritis, recurrent vomiting and gastro-oesophageal reflux (GOR). Other medical conditions result in tube-feeding because the illness reduces appetite and good nutritional status is important to reduce the degenerative progress of the disease: for example cystic fibrosis. In some cases the medical condition will prevent oral feeding from ever occurring or from being the sole source of nutrition. For others, however, the period of tube-feeding is temporary and oral feeding can begin following medical go-ahead. Some children are tube-fed for non-organic failure to thrive and in these cases oral introduction of food can begin immediately following accurate diagnosis. Though these children will not have physical incapacity for oral intake, their restricted experience can result in difficulties accepting food orally.

When an infant or child has received nutrition via a tube for a period of time significant in relation to their age, the transfer to oral feeding appears to be problematic in most cases (Jenkins and Milla 1988). An evaluation of feeding dysfunction following tube-feeding in children with chronic renal failure was carried out by Strologo *et al.* (1997). Persistent feeding problems identified were: food refusal, difficulties chewing and swallowing, and 'panic attacks' when swallowing.

Clinical experience also supports the descriptions in the literature of feeding difficulty following tube-feeding. The feeding programme for young children at Great Ormond Street Hospital for Children offers assessment and treatment for a range of feeding difficulties. An attempt to classify feeding difficulties produced some differentiation but no mutually exclusive categories indicating the complexity of these problems. Types of feeding difficulty reported included inadequate quantity eaten, selective eating, refusing to chew or swallow, slow eating and inappropriate texture for age. One third of all the children seen had experienced tube-feeding in the first six months of life and many more had experienced a period of tube-feeding at some stage in their pre-school years (Douglas and Bryon 1996). The indication is that tube-feeding is prescribed for a wide range of feeding difficulties in children with the corresponding implication that a proportion of these children will have difficulties with consequent oral intake.

Despite the wide prevalence of tube-feeding in the paediatric population and the difficulties of resuming oral feeding following medical decision to terminate tube nutrition, there is scant attention paid to this problem in the literature. There are no studies that lead to empirical hypotheses for food refusal following tube removal and few references to descriptions of the problems and treatment interventions. This chapter focuses on clinical experience of interventions following tube-feeding for children and the treatment is described by case illustration.

Why do children refuse food following tube-feeding?

It is possible to speculate why children find acceptance of oral feeding difficult following a period of tube-feeding. It is important that this question is explored as it allows more adequate understanding of the problem. Any valid areas can then form the basis of assessment for an individual child and family, which will inform appropriate intervention.

Missed critical period

Tube-feeding in infancy will restrict experience of oral feeding, but to what extent is this disruption significant for the development of feeding skills? Theories of critical periods for the acquisition of skill have been mostly dispensed with as recent studies have thrown doubt on the stage model of development and demonstrated that child development is a complex process of physical, cognitive and experiential influences. There have been few studies which have examined the development of oral-motor function following periods of tube-feeding in infants. Howver, research examining the development of sucking, swallowing and breathing in term and pre-term infants may throw light on the area. Results of these studies indicate that adequate neuromuscular coordination is more a function of gestational maturity than of post-natal sucking experience (Bu'Lock *et al.* 1990). While not directly answering the question, the suggestion is that oral-motor capability is more strongly determined centrally (i.e. neurologically) than locally via oral experience.

The notion of critical period may not have a major bearing on the infant's refusal of oral intake following tube-feeding, but does the experience of tube-feeding itself interfere with the child's developing expectations of feeding behaviour? There is some evidence that the type of feeding established in early infancy influences the child's demands for food at later stages (Wright 1988). It has been found that breast- versus bottle-fed babies differ in the amounts of feed taken at various times of the day, with breast-fed babies being more likely than the bottle-fed babies to control the amount of feed taken themselves. Tube-fed babies have no control over their intake and as such, there may be subtle, yet pervasive, effects on the infant's experience of the success of their interactions with their environment.

Experience of hunger and appetite regulation

Clinical experience indicates that parents frequently make the observation that their tube-fed infants never cry for food. Disinterest in food was reported in 63% of pre-school children referred for feeding difficulties (Douglas and Bryon 1996). Normal infants will attract carer attention by crying, exhibit restlessness and execute seeking movements toward the food (Paul and Dittrichova 1982). The nature of tube-feeding is to ensure adequate nutrition for the infant's physical size. The infant has no control over the amount of the feed nor the spacing between intake as have normal infants. It can be hypothesised that tube-fed infants do not learn to identify the physical sensations of hunger nor behaviours to signal these to their carers. In turn, the carers cease to interpret behaviours in their infant that would normally signal hunger.

In many cases tube-feeds are given according to a regimen which does not match normal appetite patterns. Often tube-feeds are prescribed to be given continuously as a drip overnight (pump-feeders for home use are widely available). The rationale here is to leave the day free for the possibility of normal appetite occurring. Some children and infants are prescribed feeds throughout the day in order to maintain adequate nutrition irrespective of natural appetite patterns. The overall result is that tube-fed babies and children do not have access to their body's physical regulation of hunger, they do not recognise the drive and they do not develop behaviours that indicate an active participation in feeding and appetite control.

Fear of food and aversive associations

All tube-fed children will have some physical disturbance of their normal alimentary processes. Many of these children will have had experience of pain and/or vomiting in association with feeding. Some will have undergone invasive medical intervention and may have chronic conditions for which such investigations will continue. On introduction of oral feeding it has been reported that disturbances of chewing and swallowing are observed (Strologo *et al.* 1997). It may be that these arise from a reluctance to accept oral food but, whatever the reason, it is almost inevitable that further failure to adequately ingest the food will maintain the aversive association.

There are other aversive associations of the experience of tube-feeding itself which are reported clinically, though not in the literature. It may be that the position of a nasogastric tube interferes with olfactory senses that affect appetite. Additionally, the experience of receiving a tube-feed via both nasogastric and gastrostomy tubes in some cases causes physical discomfort such as bloating, flatulence and hyperglycaemic symptoms. For these infants and children, receiving nutrition via any source has strong aversive associations.

Behavioural and emotional 'blocks'

Tube-feeding as an infant's main source of nutrition renders the baby passive in all aspects of the experience of feeding. The child does not learn to recognise hunger or how to act on his or her environment to satisfy a natural drive. The child misses out on a learning experience not only of having needs met but in acquiring behaviours that have a cause–effect function, which form fundamentals of communication and enable experience of human interaction. Of course, there are other areas of the child's life in which all these features can be expressed, but in respect of feeding, the child is very much 'mute'.

On a behavioural level, the child and parents have no need for a daily routine of feeding. Often in these families the tube-fed infant or child is never required to sit at a dining table or in a high chair and there is no meal-time paraphernalia associated with that child. The parents are not used to shopping and preparing food for the tube-fed child. There must be a major behavioural shift for these families to begin to incorporate the tube-fed child in their normal meal times.

On an emotional level, the effects of being a tube-fed child and of caring for a tube-fed child are no less profound. Nutritional intake during the pre-school years can generally be described as a passive process, as the concept of feeding or being fed denotes, in comparison to the term 'eating'. As mentioned, however, even neonates are not completely passive in the process and learn to affect the behaviour of others in order to have their nutritional needs met. Tube-feeding does not allow this freedom for control and it can be hypothesised that the tube-fed child's refusal of oral food is a means of initiating some control that is otherwise denied

An adult perspective may be that to be allowed oral intake following the discomfort of tube-feeding can only be positive and pleasurable. A child's perspective may be very different. To consciously open one's mouth to receive a 'foreign body' without the preparation of 'unconscious' neonatal experiences of taste, appetite regulation, drive satisfaction and trust in the meal-time behaviour and relationship of one's parents may be fraught with anxiety. Additionally, for the parents, the absence of feeding experience for their child may alter their affect and competence. There is evidence that maternal sensitivity during meal times affects the likelihood of feeding problems in the child (Sanders *et al.* 1993; Hagekull *et al.* 1997). Thus, behaviourally and emotionally, both the child and parents may have failed to develop the appropriate routines and attitudes for satisfactory oral feeding.

Experience of tube-feeding

Some case examples of referred children with a history of tube-feeding illustrate the experience of families faced with the difficulty of a child refusing oral intake when there are no longer medical reasons for maintaining tube-feeding.

Alan

Alan was referred by his gastroenterologist for refusal of oral intake. He was aged 11 months, lived with both natural parents and an older sister aged three years. Alan was born at 35 weeks gestation and was noted to have a poor suckle reflex. He refused the breast and so was bottle-fed, but this was a slow process, and he would cough and vomit throughout the feed. Each feed was a time-consuming process which became increasingly anxiety-provoking and aversive for Alan's parents as they feared he would vomit the feed. It can be suggested that feeding was also aversive for Alan with the bottle being associated with pain and vomiting. After three weeks Alan was showing no progress in weight gain and a nasogastric tube was sited. He was prescribed anti-reflux medication which reduced the size and frequency of the vomits. At the appropriate age weaning to solid foods was commenced but this restimulated the vomiting and Alan began to cry at the sight of the spoon.

Paul

Paul was referred by his nephrologist for refusal to eat orally. He was aged three years at referral and lived with both natural parents and an older sister aged five years. Paul was born with dysplastic kidneys, he had been exclusively tube-fed from birth and had received dialysis. He had received a kidney transplant at age two years and following recovery from the operation oral feeding was attempted. Paul had refused any food and would cry and gag at the sight of food intended for him.

Megan

Megan was referred by her GP for refusal of oral solids and liquids. Megan was aged 19 months and lived with both her natural parents; she was an only child. Megan was born full-term by normal delivery but had meconium aspiration; she spent one week in the special care baby unit where she was nasogastrically tube-fed. Megan was then discharged home on a mixture of breast- and bottle-feeding, but she was slow to feed and did not gain weight. At 18 days she began vomiting her feeds; investigations revealed pyloric stenosis and she underwent corrective surgery. At four months of age Megan was readmitted to hospital for food refusal and nasogastric tube-feeding recommenced. The ensuing months were marked by a constant attempt to introduce oral feeding to no avail. Meal times had become aversive for her parents and were more or less abandoned in favour of total tube-feeding. Megan would refuse to open her mouth for the spoon.

For all three families, though the reasons for commencement of tube-feeding were different, the presenting problems were the same. The children had initial physical difficulties with food digestion and consequent adequate weight gain. There had been a history of vomiting with oral intake. Attempts to establish an effective oral feeding pattern had failed, becoming aversive and anxiety-provoking for parents and child. Tube-feeding had solved the weight gain problem and removed troublesome meal times from the households. For all three families it had been a medical decision to start oral feeding and it must be acknowledged that for the families tube-feeding had its advantages.

Management of change from tube to oral feeding

To illustrate the assessment and intervention for introduction of oral intake to a tube-fed child one of the above cases is described in detail.

Alan – initial assessment

A videotape was made of a meal time with Alan being offered age-appropriate solid foods by his mother, who was the major carer. It was noted that his mother chose appropriate food, texture, portion size and utensils for his developmental age. This indicated that she was aware of her son's level and of normal feeding expectations despite lack of feeding experience with Alan. She placed the bowl of food near to Alan and he touched the food tentatively. Alan held an empty spoon. Alan's mother was wary of putting a spoon loaded with food to Alan's mouth in case it stimulated a vomit. She also kept control of the bowl. Alan gagged when his mother loaded a spoon with food even though she had not offered it to him.

It was clear that although Alan's mother was trying hard to maintain a friendly atmosphere, the interaction was strained and Alan showed increasing signs of distress the longer he was sat near to the food. Same-age peers with no history of food refusal would have grabbed the bowl, touched the food, attempted to load a spoon themselves and put it to mouth, and they may have been simultaneously gnawing on some finger foods.

Intervention 1

The aims were to enable pleasurable meal times, to gain the parents' trust and faith in the intervention, and to instigate change to the current meal times. The initial goals were to support the friendly atmosphere seen in the video assessment. Alan's mother was given positive feedback and discussions were around acknowledgement of the strain of meal times and reasons why they were not relaxed. It was important to listen to and accept the parental need for a slow pace of change. They had to be allowed some jurisdiction as parents and have the difficult feeding history appreciated. Behavioural changes took place that involved instigating regular family meal times, which included Alan. Alan was to be presented with food of a very runny texture. His parents were to play with the food and show him how they eat; utensils were to be present but no spoons should be loaded for Alan.

A programme of desensitisation to solid food was begun. Puréed food was first placed on mother's finger and dabbed around the plate and increasingly closer to Alan, stopping at the moment of distress. Purée was then placed on a finger food and again placed nearer to Alan until he would hold the finger food himself. His mother's empty finger was then moved increasingly towards Alan's mouth in a playful manner but at a meal time. Alan then began to accept an empty spoon to his mouth, held by himself, then an empty spoon held by his parents. These steps took several weeks and did not progress smoothly through a hierarchy but moved backwards and forwards depending on the emotional state of all concerned.

Changes to meal times

Changes occurring during these initial interventions were as follows: Alan began to suck runny purée off his own fingers and finger foods. Alan was beginning to show interest in other people eating, particularly his sister. Alan then began accepting a spoon dipped in purée from his sister. He then began to accept a trainer beaker of water and would take about two sips per day. The range of food that his parents had thought to offer him increased. Alan was beginning to take tastes more willingly of a range of foods. The next break-through was that Alan allowed his mother to touch his lips with gravy on her finger. Overall, Alan's interest in food and meal times and his willingness to let his mother and sister offer food without stimulating distress or vomiting increased his mother's confidence and motivated her to offer more food. The atmosphere at meal times became less strained and his parents even began to look forward to breakthroughs. Alan's parents had begun to change their perception of him from non-eater (tube-reliant) to eater.

Intervention 2

Alan had begun to accept minute amounts of food orally but still received all his nutrition via a tube. Alan had not experienced hunger or appetite, though he was beginning to experience positive meal times. A goal now was to stimulate hunger and this would involve reducing tube-feeds. At this stage it was essential to consult with his gastroenterologist and dietician and to clarify a plan of action with agreement of all concerned.

The plan was first to establish that his weight was satisfactory and there was some weight to 'play with'. In some cases it may be necessary to increase tube-feeds to put up the child's weight before any reduction can begin. Tube-feeds were reduced by a small amount for two consecutive days then returned to their original amount. This pace satisfied his parent's need to maintain the weight gain that they had struggled for. Any changes in the quantity of oral food Alan consumed were noted. Tube-feeds were then reduced for longer time periods. There was an initial weight loss that his parents had been expecting, so it was easier to handle. There was a slower, but noticeable increase in Alan's oral intake of both solid foods and water. This pattern proceeded with gradually longer periods of time at reduced tube-feeds. Alan's parents received regular support and his weight was monitored.

Final changes

Alan began to accept thicker textures. Vomiting occurred on occasions during this phase, but gradually reduced. Alan began eating more finger foods of bite-dissolve texture. The quantity of oral intake increased and eventually all tube-feeds stopped. Weight gain was maintained without tube-feeding. It took 12 months from referral to removal of the nasogastric tube with fortnightly appointments. Alan was then monitored much less frequently for a further year.

Summary of intervention for children who are tube-fed

Meal times

- regular meal times (with the family)
- purée and bite-dissolve finger foods (irrespective of age of child) are within reach of the child
- no pressure to eat

- meal times of short duration
- playful atmosphere.

Desensitisation

- to presence of food
- to presence of utensils
- to dipped utensils (in purée)
- to dipped finger foods
- to dipped fingers
- to approach of fingers to face
- to approach of food to face
- encouragement of self-feeding.

Tube-feeds

- collaborate with other involved medical professionals
- ensure have weight to play with
- reduce tube-feeds
- there will be an initial weight loss
- there will be an initial mismatch between hunger and eating
- then a gradual catch up so oral intake increases.

This summary provides the skeleton of a behavioural intervention for introduction of oral feeding to pre-school children who are refusing food. It is
important to remember that causes and maintenance of food refusal can be
multifactorial and thorough assessment is essential with eventual interventions being tailored to the individual child and family (Harris 1993).

Conclusions

Prolonged or significant tube-feeding in the pre-school years can disrupt
natural experiences of feeding for the child and parents to the extent that
oral feeding cannot be successfully begun or resumed without professional
intervention. Possible reasons why oral feeding may be refused in these
children have been described and indicate the need for thorough assessment
and multilevel intervention.

The typical behavioural intervention for food refusal following tube-feeding
described here incorporated three basic levels: changes to the meal-time
structure, desensitisation of the child to the anxiety-provoking food and

reduction of tube-feeding. Although this particular intervention has not been subjected to experimental evaluation, similar behavioural interventions for feeding difficulties in pre-school children have also been successful (O'Brien *et al.* 1991; Munk and Repp 1994). Prospective evaluation of such interventions will add greatly to clinical practice for food refusal in tube-fed young children.

References

Bu'Lock F, Woolridge MW and Baum JD (1990) Development of co-ordination of sucking, swallowing and breathing: ultrasound study of term and preterm infants. *Developmental Medicine and Child Neurology.* **32**(8): 669–78.

Douglas JE and Bryon M (1996) Interview data on severe behavioural eating difficulties in young children. *Archives of Disease in Childhood.* **75**: 304–8.

Hagekull B, Bohlin G and Rydell AM (1997) Maternal sensitivity, infant temperament and the development of early feeding problems. *Infant Mental Health Journal.* **18**(1): 92–106.

Harris G (1993) Feeding problems and their treatment. In: I St James, G Harris and D Messer (eds) *Infant Crying, Feeding and Sleeping: development, problems and treatments*, pp 118–32. Harvester Wheatsheaf, London.

Jenkins J and Milla P (1988) Feeding problems and failure to thrive. In: N Richman, R Lansdown (eds) *Problems of Pre-school Children*, pp 151–72. John Wiley, Chichester.

Lindberg L, Bohlin G and Hagekull B (1991) Early feeding problems in a normal population. *International Journal of Eating Disorders.* **10**(4): 395–405.

Linscheid TR, Budd KS and Rasnake LK (1995) Pediatric feeding disorders. In: MC Roberts (ed) *Handbook of Pediatric Psychology* (2e). Guilford Press, New York.

Munk DD and Repp AC (1994) Behavioural assessment of feeding problems of individuals with severe disabilities. Special issue: Functional analysis approaches to behavioural assessment and treatment. *Journal of Applied Behaviour Analysis.* **27**(2): 241–50.

O'Brien S, Repp AC, Williams GE and Christopherson ER (1991) Pediatric feeding disorders. Special issue: Current perspectives in the diagnosis, assessment and treatment of child and adolescent disorders. *Behaviour Modification.* **15**(3): 194–418.

Paul K and Dittrichova J (1982) Feeding behaviour in newborns. *Activitas Nervosa Superior.* **24**(3): 131–2.

Reau NR, Senturia YD, Lebailly SA and Christoffel KK (1996) Infant and toddler feeding patterns and problems. Normative data and a new direction. *Journal of Developmental and Behavioral Pediatrics.* **17**(3): 149–53.

Sanders MR, Patel RK, le Grice B and Shepherd RW (1993) Children with persistent feeding difficulties: an observational analysis of the feeding interactions of problem and non-problem eaters. *Health Psychology*. **12**(1): 64–73.

Strologo LD, Principato F, Sinibaldi D, Appiani AC, Terzi F, Dartois AM and Rizzoni G (1997) Feeding dysfunction in infants with severe chronic renal failure after long-term nasogastric tube-feeding. *Pediatric Nephrology*. **11**: 84–6.

Wright P (1988) Learning experiences in feeding behaviour during infancy. 31st Annual Conference of the Society for Psychosomatic Research. *Journal of Psychosomatic Research*. **32**(6): 613–19.

CHAPTER 13

Feeding problems in children with chronic illness

Anthony Schwartz

Introduction

This chapter outlines psychological issues and approaches to managing feeding problems in children who have chronic and life-threatening illnesses. As such, it takes into consideration developmental issues, family and physical health factors, consultation and liaison aspects, and ends with treatment frameworks for good practice. Theoretical approaches to working with children, carers, professionals and the medical–social systems implicated in treatment are highlighted (e.g. individual therapeutic approaches, application of systemic work and professional training). It is hoped that this will give the reader an overview of the multiple and complex 'psychological' roles in a problem area that is many-layered and multidimensional. Ultimately the aim is to encourage both learning and sharing in a field that needs to use its resources to develop creative solutions.

Psychological approaches to feeding difficulties need to be seen in the context of paediatric care, within the discipline of paediatric psychology. It is necessary to look at the problem of paediatric chronic illness, feeding problems and their management by examining the concerns at three levels. First, there are child influences (within and around the child); second, the family influences; and third, the interface of the child–professional system. Only once there has been an agreed focus and plan taking into account interdisciplinary working can clinical applications and techniques be implemented. It is my aim to highlight this process, acknowledging the unique abilities and roles of all members of the treatment team, including the child, family and health professionals.

Psychological and social dimensions in both the course and treatment of a chronic illness are important fields of investigation. La Greca and Varni (1993) call for research to focus on psychosocial and developmental factors that contribute to the treatment of paediatric conditions. Issues for children with chronic diseases impact on the child, the family and the health carers, often with multiple hospital admissions and numerous treatments. Unfortunately, Drotar (1997) points out that most psychological research on paediatric chronic illness has focused primarily on description of associated psychosocial problems rather than on interventions to reduce these. This criticism can be equally applied to feeding problems in children with chronic illness. The aim of this chapter is to consolidate some of the evidence on interventions so as to start redressing that imbalance.

The context of feeding problems in chronic illness

Technically, medicine has helped to prolong life and to treat children who might previously have died. With these technological advances comes the need for psychological interventions to assist with the management of the child's ongoing treatment. Children with kidney disease, cystic fibrosis, liver disease and cancers are all surviving well into adulthood, with a total prevalence of children with chronic conditions of 10% (Fielding 1985). Pless and Roghmann (1971) quote a prevalence figure of between 10 and 20%, based on parental report using a broad definition of chronic illness.

Childhood eating disorders are relatively rare in school-age children (Altman and Lock 1997), although feeding problems are quite common especially where there are other coexisting illnesses. Baer (1997) cites figures of between 10 and 42% for feeding problems in children with chronic illness, such as kidney conditions, liver disease, inflammatory bowel syndromes, human immunodeficiency virus infection, cystic fibrosis, diabetes, cancer, phenylketonuria, neurological problems and allergies. However, in maintaining their lives, other problems need to be addressed. Primary to life-sustenance is the provision of food, the importance of eating and eating sufficient of the right foodstuffs. If these natural processes are the subject of intense focus and scrutiny, it can lead to heightened awareness, anxiety and conflict for children, families and healthcare staff.

Children with chronic conditions are involved in many professional systems. Specific difficulties can arise because of the complex matrices of professionals and interventions, both for the individual child and family and for the professionals. Within this group of children with chronic conditions, feeding problems may be viewed as occurring along a continuum, with children at the most severe end being maintained on nasogastric tube-feeding for years. As emphasised by Baer and Harris (1997) a child may have any combination of problems with an even greater number of health professionals being implicated in their treatment. This may raise inter-professional and communication difficulties as the network may include community and acute paediatrics, dental services, dietetics, community paediatric nursing, speech therapy, occupational therapy and psychological services. The list may seem endless, and Woody (1990) describes the inclusion of a paediatric neurologist perspective in feeding disorders. Working with a number of professionals and agencies has vast implications, with professionals likely to adopt contrasting positions which affect clinical effectiveness (Dale 1996).

Where children have a concurrent illness alongside a feeding problem this may be considered to be a 'complex-case scenario'. There are likely to be heightened feelings underpinned by experience, not the least of which are living with a chronic condition and dealing with various medical and nursing treatments and interventions. It may be suggested that this constellation of feeding problems within chronic or life-threatening illnesses adds considerable intensity for the child, the family and the healthcare professionals involved.

Normal eating and people in exceptional circumstances

There are immediate problems in defining what may be considered to be 'normal eating' (Shepherd *et al.* 1971). Where the child has been diagnosed as having a clear organic condition general child management and feeding can be affected. However, anxiety about feeding seems to 'go with the territory' of early child-rearing. Wardley *et al.* (1997) make the point that an array of symptoms occur in babies, which are associated with or ascribed to feeding or digestive processes. These cause parents emotional concern and can lead to emotional disturbances and distortion of the parent–child relationship (*see* Chapters 4 and 8). Most psychologists see only those children whose parents have sought help with general feeding problems. When feeding problems are of deeper concern, there is usually a referral from a healthcare professional who is worried about a child's condition. Psychological assessment would normally occur following referral by a health visitor, nurse, general practitioner or paediatrician. A good psychological and medical screening needs to be undertaken to differentiate between a feeding problem, an acute or chronic illness, or when a child's refusal to eat is related to unrealistic parental expectations. Leung and Robson (1994) support the provision of psychological input in all the above, beginning with reassurance and counselling and possibly later working at a deeper and more complex level if the assessment, formulation and therapy undertaken indicate this would be beneficial. Such considerations should take into account evidence-based practice.

Complicating the issue of comparing literature is the problem of definition of feeding problems in children, as described in the introduction. Widely disparate estimates of feeding problems seem to occur because there is little chance of evaluating and comparing the data which are based on different types of problem description and severity. One enters a maze of problem classification and categorisation, with professionals using different epistemological frameworks. The most common is the 'medical model', which emphasises differential diagnosis and assessment through a process of convergent thinking, whereas psychological formulations look at more lateral and divergent problem solving. There are potential problems when discrepancies in evaluation occur with problems of psychological problem description and formulation in contrast to psychiatric nosology and criteria, and frequently elements of each of the above. However, it would not be fair to say that feeding problems are a psychiatric problem with all that is associated with such labelling. Rather, children with chronic illnesses and feeding problems remain very much 'ordinary people in exceptional circumstances' (Eiser 1990). Bradford (1997) confirms that most children do not have mental health problems, and questions whether issues of children's adjustment should be approached using mental health and psychiatric categorisation, pointing out that this can be unnecessarily restricting.

Archer *et al.* (1991) accept that the assessment and treatment of these behaviours have been highly variable, reflecting the number of disciplines involved and the lack of a clear conceptual framework and classification system within which to view the problems. Nevertheless, the *International Classification of Diseases*, 10th Revision (WHO 1992) criteria require that a feeding disorder in infancy or childhood 'generally involves refusal of food or extreme faddiness'.

Concerns, anxiety, depression and other emotional factors are considered to affect the feeding process of otherwise healthy children. How much more likely is this when a child has a chronic or life-threatening illness? Hence the importance of management of emotional factors associated with feeding and chronic illness. It is necessary to be fully aware of the literature and to understand general child development with its transitions and emotional and behavioural concomitants from a number of theoretical perspectives as well as their critiques (Carey 1985; Erikson 1980; Piaget 1976). Although one needs to pay attention to the child's age and stage of development, research on developmental aspects will not be covered here other than to acknowledge this as important. Inter-relationship factors between the child and parent, and parental emotional issues, have been raised in some of the other chapters and will be reviewed briefly below in terms of how they affect the feeding process.

There are very few studies on the effects of parental eating attitudes and behaviours on the development of children's feeding patterns. However, Hellin and Waller (1992) found that maternal mood was associated with feeding problems. There was an association between women with higher anxiety reporting more problems with infants' feeding behaviours and giving up breast-feeding sooner than non-anxious mothers. Depressed mothers were found to have more problems with breast-feeding. Although these links are not evidence of causality, it would be useful to have further evidence of intervention studies with women found to have mood-related issues early in pregnancy. There are implications for psychological support and work to be done regarding self-efficacy, self-confidence and cognitive schemas for women early on in pregnancy to prevent the formation of a vicious cycle of mood and feeding disturbance, if the results of this study can be generalised. The issue of long-term follow-up remains, and the question arises whether these initial feeding problems develop into more pervasive problems around eating owing to an early problem template having been established.

Stein *et al.* (1995) concluded that a link exists between disturbed maternal eating habits and attitudes. It reinforces the need to engage in a comprehensive assessment interview with parents, which should include careful and sensitive questioning about the parents' own eating habits and attitudes. This is essential to good psychological practice. Additionally, Evans and le Grange (1995) found that 'eating-disordered mothers' schedule-fed their babies, whereas those without eating problems fed their babies on demand. Recommendations for further good practice emerging from this study highlight the need for careful instruction and support for mothers with eating problems of their own. The question of how maternal characteristics influence feeding is important. It is, nevertheless, necessary to keep in mind an interactional perspective with the individual characteristics of the child as co-determining factors in development and parenting.

It is important to understand the process of establishing 'normal' eating habits and how these may be affected when individual children are struggling with chronic and life-threatening conditions, i.e. living under exceptional circumstances.

Feeding difficulties associated with chronic illness

Studies of children in hospital with chronic illness have indicated a high prevalence of malnutrition (Wardley *et al.* 1997). Malnutrition has effects on the child's resilience and has potentially serious consequences for all body systems. As a result, nutritional interventions are used to supplement calorific intake and alter the natural history of the disease. Linked with these specific treatments come anxieties about how and when to intervene, fears about invasive procedures, worry about whether the child is gaining sufficient weight, issues of control, and problems in managing treatment, all of which have psychological relevance. Archer *et al.* (1991) clearly link elements in a vicious cycle by which professionals' therapeutic decisions to increase the frequency of feeding or provide special diets result in parental worry or fear about nutritional intake, which makes for a functional feeding problem where feeding behaviours and management are affected.

Feeding problems associated with chronic illness can be similar to those found in the general population, e.g. poor appetite, food faddiness or selectivity, taking a long time to eat, not seeking food at all, food refusal, gagging and vomiting.

What will be described now are specific forms of intervention where there are clear psychological issues to be dealt with.

Enteral nutrition

Artificial feeding reduces food to its barest essential, that of nourishing the patient, and excludes the social dimensions, cultural aspects and physical sensations that normally go with eating (Padilla and Grant 1985). Psychological considerations surrounding this method may be linked to the timing (i.e. when this form of feeding is instituted), to the treatment procedure itself (i.e. insertion or passing of the tube) and to the consequences of long-term use of this means (i.e. inability to take oral feeds subsequently). Decisions to institute nasogastric feeding may be made where there have been unsuccessful attempts at providing sufficient nutrition orally. Frustration on the part of parents when a child is not taking adequate food orally may lead to an aversive parent–child feeding milieu. Psychological involvement may support a medical intervention or might focus on management of the vicious cycle of anxiety and dysfunctional interaction. There is also often a need for support to be given to the parents regarding the benefits of this form of treatment. Some of these issues are psychologically critical as they affect management, adherence and emotional concerns for both individuals and families.

Invasive procedures have been shown to be some of the most feared aspects for children undergoing medical treatment (Ross and Ross 1988). The management of distress, fear and pain in the paediatric setting has been cited as an area for specific psychological applications (Schwartz and Mercer 1998). Practical psychological help is useful in the form of distraction, relaxation and reframing the experience of the nasogastric tube insertion, as is highlighted in a short case example.

> *Case example 1: Nicky, a 10-year-old girl, was seen by individual nurses in the paediatric community nursing team to help pass her nasogastric tube. Sessions often lasted for up to three hours. Nicky's mother was concerned about her daughter and often interrupted the*

process to ask how Nicky was feeling about the procedure. She also emphasised to the professionals how difficult it was to perform, and how worried Nicky was about the procedure. As a result, sessions were highly emotionally charged. Following discussion at a case management meeting, it was decided to focus on what had made interventions successful in the past. Assisting Nicky's mother to manage her anxiety was suggested. Following distraction for both Nicky and her mother (which included mother being asked to focus on another activity such as making coffee) the level of anxiety diminished and a cycle of positive experiences was started. The major benefit meant that the passing of the tube took a few minutes rather than a few hours.

Vomiting and nausea

Medical treatment advances have led to the control of vomiting and nausea in patients undergoing cancer chemotherapy. However, with other conditions there remain concerns about nausea as a side effect of treatment (e.g. haemodialysis) or as a result of acute anxiety. Problems such as habitual reflex vomiting have been shown to benefit from psychological approaches (Sokel *et al.* 1991), focusing on helping the young person to achieve gradual control over the symptom (e.g. using relaxation and guided imagery). These authors also mention shaping of behaviour by positive reinforcement of food retention and 'time-out' for vomiting as alternative approaches to managing vomiting. An example of work which began with multidisciplinary role confusion in managing a conditioned anxiety state is described below.

> *Case example 2: James, a young man of 17 years old with a long history of feeding problems, was hospitalised for a number of months on the paediatric ward. As a person with some learning difficulties, he had been struggling at school for a considerable period, although there had been no special educational provision. On the ward James had been found to be very selective with his eating habits and frequently went to the toilet immediately following meals. He expressed feeling anxious and tense, and was under pressure to 'eat properly'. The consultant paediatrician referred James to a child and adolescent psychiatry service. Since this service only offers input to young people up to the age of 16 years, it was suggested that James be referred to an adult psychiatry eating disorder service. Following assessment by the psychiatrist, who considered that he did not have an eating disorder, it was suggested that he be referred to a learning disabilities service. Unfortunately, there was some confusion about*

the referral and action to be undertaken. As a result the consultant paediatrician discussed this with the paediatric psychologist following a case management meeting on the paediatric ward. Until this point this young man had been in hospital for three months. Ongoing work was initiated with paediatric psychology involvement and James was discharged after a graded programme to manage his anxiety and to reintegrate him into the home and school environments. Interventions were continued on an outpatient basis, with James developing increased social and educational skills. His nausea and vomiting stopped, and his eating behaviours were of no concern upon follow-up after one year.

Nutritional deficits

Medical management of nutritional deficits, absorption problems and anatomical changes such as anorexia in chronic conditions are usually through the use of nasal-oesophageal feeding tubes or hyperalimentation where nutrients are delivered directly into the blood. There is limited published research on behavioural treatments for anorexia (rather than anorexia nervosa) in children with chronic illness. One study (Cairns and Altman 1979) describes the use of positive social reinforcement, access to play activities and a token system to reverse weight loss in paediatric oncology. Other researchers comment on the importance of management of anorexia but fail to include any psychological frameworks (Ravelli 1995). Emphasis appears to be on the usefulness of physical treatments to deal with these problems (Warady *et al.* 1990), although where there are learned food aversions, behavioural strategies have been shown to be effective (Hoch *et al.* 1994; O'Brien *et al.* 1991) as have hypnobehavioural approaches (Culbert *et al.* 1996). In addition, where there are high states of anxiety, for example in swallowing disorders, use of biofeedback and psycho-physiological methods can be usefully applied.

Themes of problems for children with chronic illness

As suggested earlier, demarcating difficulties into 'medical' versus 'psychological' categories is not particularly helpful in the process of treatment. The need is for a holistic formulation of the child within the biological, psychological and social context, using ideas from health psychology and systemic theory (Bradford 1997). However, one might suggest that there is practical use in retaining a 'medical condition' framework, since we frequently encounter this diagnostic division first when being presented with a feeding difficulty in a child with a concomitant illness. Research supports the contention that children with chronic illness are at greater risk for feeding problems (Culbert *et al.* 1996). There is meagre information on percentages of children with feeding problems by selected medical diagnosis with only one author (Baer 1997) quoting prevalence figures collated from a specific geographical region. What follows are descriptions of feeding issues in the most commonly presenting conditions in the paediatric psychology context. It is not meant to be an exhaustive exemplar of work in this field, but it is aimed at highlighting some pertinent management problems.

Cancer

Overt malnutrition is found in children with cancer (Wardley *et al.* 1997). The aetiology of this has been described as children having a lack of appetite, psychological factors such as learned food aversions, malabsorption, excess nutrient loss and increased caloric demands as a result of tumours (van Eys 1979). Early effects of treatment may affect adequate intake with disturbances in taste, changes in food preference, nausea and vomiting (Eiser 1998), and Kelly (1986) refers to relaxation techniques to improve patients' intake. Useful psychological interventions with learned food aversions are behavioural and cognitive strategies (Rickhard *et al.* 1986). Research has highlighted non-medical treatment for cancer-related anorexia (Cairns and Altman 1979) through the use of positive reinforcement. Epston (1994) describes a case study from a family systems perspective using hypnosis for management of chemotherapy-related appetite loss. More recently, Zeltzer *et al.* (1996), in a seven site study, showed that eating problems occur in siblings of children with cancer. Yet these authors confirm that healthcare interventions in siblings are reduced in comparison to other children. They recommend that psychologists should not forget the needs of siblings and include questions about the other children and their eating habits when meeting with the family of children with chronic and life-threatening conditions. This is additional to special work helping children whose siblings have cancer in oncology units at specialist children's hospitals (Balen *et al.* 1998).

Cystic fibrosis

As a result of the number of physical treatments required and the widely held belief that higher calorific intake and added weight may act as a buffer against infection, feeding issues are in the forefront when children have cystic fibrosis.

Excessive focus on food, feeding and weight gain can lead to abnormal feeding patterns and negative feeding behaviour, with 37% of children over a year old with cystic fibrosis experiencing feeding difficulties (MacDonald 1996). Pearson *et al.* (1991) found that youngsters aged eight to 15 years were significantly more likely to have eating disturbances in the form of resisting food, being preoccupied with food and using food as a control issue than an older group aged 16 to 40 years. The latter groups were found to have more depressed and anxious symptoms. MacDonald (1996) indicates that problems may include prolonged meal times, vomiting and gagging, force-feeding, constant parental nagging and food refusal and suggests that help from a psychologist with an interest in feeding problems is invaluable. Parental anxiety about food, acute infections and frequent disruptions as a result of hospital admissions may all affect the home atmosphere and interactions. This may be manifest in tense and upsetting meal times with parents pressing food on to a child, giving increased attention through coaxing or removal from the feeding situation, all of which serve to maintain a child's avoidance (Singer *et al.* 1991). They also found that mothers' fear that their child would die affected their meal-time interactions with their child.

Sanders *et al.* (1997) found that parents of cystic fibrosis children reported more disruption, emphasised behaviour management problems and cited lower marital satisfaction. Problems associated with growth abnormalities were also in evidence. However, observational data did not indicate that these children were significantly different in meal-time behaviours. This has implications for psychological practice around meal times, which are pressured times for parents who are trying to ensure their child receives adequate nutrition. They suggest that interventions would need to be at three levels: the first deals with how to promote dietary compliance (e.g. through learning non-aversive parental management strategies and having guidelines about optimal instruction giving). The second addresses parental feelings on inadequacy, helplessness and uncertainty about how to cope with their child's illness, as well as expectations about the dietary intake needed. Third, programmes would need to focus on family distress and the inter-relationships between the parents.

Diabetes

Emphasis on diet and eating in diabetes care, along with concerns about weight, may be considered to make young people vulnerable to eating problems. Pollock *et al.* (1995) found that 11.4% had at some stage had a period of eating problems. The most significant finding was that the diagnosis of eating disorder was linked to the youngster having other mental health problems. It was suggested that if young people with diabetes have eating problems, it is necessary to check if they have any other psychological problems as well. A further study on adolescents with diabetes mellitus (Neumark-Sztainer *et al.* 1996) found increased disordered eating (e.g. binge eating and purging) among adolescents with diabetes when compared to normal controls. The study was based on a self-report questionnaire to a community sample, with no confirmation of diagnosis of diabetic status, and the authors suggest that interviews might have been preferable so as to examine diabetic treatment and problems associated with the condition.

Human immunodeficiency virus (HIV)

There have been few studies on feeding problems in children with HIV and yet there are often many physical signs associated with the condition (e.g. symptoms of diarrhoea, weight loss, poor growth and developmental weakness). Melvin *et al.* (1997) emphasise that poor underlying nutrition threatens physical and psychological development. In addition, dealing with feeding-related aspects places a burden of time and effort on carers who may have their own HIV-related problems. Developmental considerations to be taken into account include the difficult period in transition from milk to solid food, which requires more energy, as well as sophisticated chewing and swallowing movements. In their study, cultural issues were implicated, with the group being of African background, where differences in weaning practices and conflicts over traditional foods versus Western 'fast' foods were evident. Other aspects include parental pressure on the child to eat, which serves to enhance negative meal-time behaviours.

Renal failure

Types of feeding problems associated with chronic kidney disease include reduced appetite, gastro-oesophageal reflux (GOR), nausea, vomiting and anorexia (Ravelli 1995; Sadowski *et al.* 1993; Strologo *et al.* 1997) all of which play a major role in growth failure often found in this group of young people. A recent study by Douglas *et al.* (1998) has shown that children's severe eating problems dramatically improved following kidney transplantation. Despite the small sample size and retrospective nature of the study, the conclusions are helpful. It also suggests that early nasogastric feeding does not affect transfer to total oral intake. The transition is likely to have been made easier by there having been less anxiety around feeding, which reinforces an earlier study (Douglas 1995) that by not having been force-fed or made to eat, children had not experienced early aversive learning.

Guidelines for good practice

General issues common to chronic conditions raised earlier in the chapter include anxiety and phobic responses, attachment, control and separation issues, listlessness, despair and depression. Throughout the chapter reference has been made to the significant role of psychological practice in the management and treatment of feeding problems overall.

The practitioner needs to know medical interventions and common problems associated with the chronic and life-threatening conditions as a whole, but more specifically and importantly should be familiar with particular medical conditions and their implications, both physically and psychologically. The need to consider the mutually influencing individual and system effects, with the impact this has on collaboration and inter-professional working, has already been looked at in Chapter 7.

Practice would indicate that psychological management of feeding problems should comprise both an 'individual perspective' and a 'metaview'. Individual focus may encompass behavioural, cognitive and psychodynamic frameworks, and an overarching perspective can be taken by using family and systemic approaches. Kendall and Norton-Ford (1982) clearly set out the need for proper assessment, problem formulation, treatment and evaluation of the approach used.

Good practice

The quintessential question concerns application of theory to develop coherent practice. Psychological assessment would normally occur following referral from a parent, health visitor, nurse, general practitioner or paediatrician.

Good practice guidelines for children with complicated conditions have not been formally published, although research has brought some issues into sharp relief. Tawfik *et al.* (1997), in their discussion on use of gastrostomy, comment that a multidisciplinary team approach, such as a specialist feeding clinic, contributes to the successful management of complex feeding problems. The study by Babbitt *et al.* (1994) adds weight to the multidisciplinary approach as does the review by O'Brien *et al.* (1991). The use of a 'transdisciplinary team', where multiple professionals are committed to work, teach and learn together across discipline boundaries (Wooster *et al.* 1998), further supports teamwork in dealing with paediatric feeding problems. These authors offer examples of case studies which show the advantages of using a transdisciplinary team in the evaluation and treatment of feeding problems. In their approach they actively promote the inclusion and participation of the family as 'the most vital member of the team'.

Linscheid (1998) emphasises competence, in that for a child with a known medical problem, it is necessary to have a working knowledge of the normal course of the disease and its treatment. In addition it is important for the psychologist to have a close working relationship with competent medical personnel.

Assessment of feeding behaviour across a variety of 'environments' (e.g. caretaker, texture of food, type of food, order of food, position, attention) is considered to be crucial (Kerwin and Berkowitz 1996). This may identify information that may help in the treatment. Kerwin and Berkowitz also contend that there should be a focus on other aspects, such as the parental functioning and interactions with the child.

Regarding children of mothers with anorexia nervosa, it is recommended that all children of mothers with such a disorder be investigated and that treatment involves the whole family, in addition to work with the mother, which should include advice on nutritional requirements of growing children (Russell *et al.* 1998).

Budd *et al.* (1992) in their study of 50 families of young children with feeding problems found that different clinical services are needed depending on the nature of the feeding problem. Developmental delays that necessitate long-term care often accompany organically based problems, with parental emotional distress being high for this group. This means that their emotional adjustment needs to be considered.

In working with parents of chronically ill children, Knafl *et al.* (1992) consider essential professional skills to be the ability to provide technically competent services, communicate with families, participate as an effective team member, be sensitive to ethical issues and conceptualise problems in ecological terms.

In their review on chronic illnesses, Elander and Midence (1997) comment on training and research implications in this specific field, including training of other professionals, which is an effective way of stretching limited resources. However, the others involved need supervision and support from a psychological perspective, especially in complex conditions such as feeding problems in chronic illness populations.

Constant evaluation of practice is needed to build up a research literature on effective management in line with the current national focus on clinical effectiveness and evidence-based medicine. Evaluation of practice and committing the findings to paper for peer audit and review is one step to improving research output in this area.

For maximum impact of individual practitioners' working it may be helpful to consider ways of improved training and awareness-raising among professionals as well as parents, with, for example, the facilitation of parent training (Werle *et al.* 1993). Periodic reviews and opportunities to summarise and reflect on the current situation and treatments all need time and require evaluation to see whether the aims of interventions are being achieved. It may be considered helpful to 'map out' the position in which the child, family and professionals with a long-term illness and feeding problems find themselves, and to take into consideration the beliefs and views of all concerned (*see* Figure 13.1). A useful method for doing this arises from personal construct psychology (Kelly 1955) and has been presented in the context of 'fit' between professionals where there are treatment adherence problems (Schwartz 1997). This model can be applied quite easily in the feeding context.

Consideration of individual practitioner skills and acknowledgement of the boundaries to competence need to be weighed up against the need to intervene to the best of one's ability based on experience and training. Where some interventions may seem to be more classical 'clinical psychology' skills than others (e.g. generic counselling) we need to accept that they will be done differently when undertaken by different professionals.

To conclude this chapter, it is anticipated that the outline of good practice will serve to consolidate the main themes and act as a mental checklist. Good practice would be underpinned by, among other things:

- the awareness that the feeding problem does not 'stand alone' but is intricately associated with the contextual factors and the child's chronic condition
- communication and contact between professionals involved are essential to the assessment, formulation and development of a comprehensive treatment plan
- interdisciplinary practices, applications and techniques need to be clear
- individual, family and systems level consultation, liaison and practice should occur, which may include local professionals and agencies (e.g. different directorates, trusts and voluntary bodies) and national networking (e.g. with tertiary referral centres)
- acknowledgement that each professional's perspective, together with those of the family and child, should be taken 'as parts which make up the whole picture'
- expect conflicting positions to be taken and make use of 'supervision' and opportunities for reflection and the adoption of a 'metastance' by someone not closely involved in the family–professional system
- gain experience and practice in using a number of strategies and techniques for working with complex problems (e.g. cognitive strategies such as 'reframing', positive reinforcement) in addition to general 'tools of the trade'
- make certain that there is ongoing training and enthusiasm to develop new and creative approaches for work in this field (it can be 'infectious')

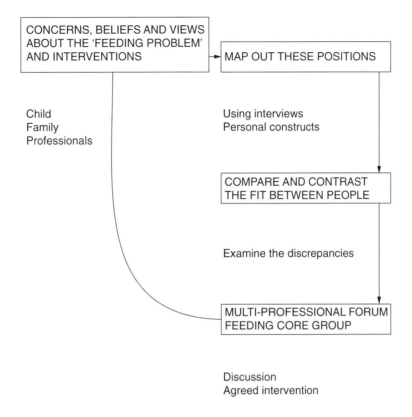

Figure 13.1: Method for evaluating whether the aims of interventions are being achieved.

- consider the needs of the family (e.g. for practical support, exploration of emotional issues for parents/relatives)
- use of feedback cycles to assess interventions and consider the 'fit' of views and constructs between participants as regards the diverse inputs
- constant evaluation of practice is needed to build up a research literature on effective management so as to add to current research in this important area.

References

Altman TM and Lock J (1997) Eating disorders. In: H Steiner (ed) *Treating School-age Children*. Jossey-Bass Publishers, San Francisco.

Archer LA, Rosenbaum PL and Steiner DL (1991) The children's eating behavior inventory: reliability and validity results. *Journal of Pediatric Psychology*. **16**: 629–42.

Babbitt RL, Hoch TA, Coe DA *et al.* (1994) Behavioural assessment and treatment of paediatric feeding disorders. *Development and Behavioral Pediatrics*. **15**: 278–91.

Baer MT (1997) Nutrition services for children with disabilities and chronic illness. In: HM Wallace, RF Biehl, JC MacQueen and JA Blackburn (eds) *Mosby's Resource Guide to Children with Disabilities and Chronic Illness*. Mosby, St Louis.

Baer MT and Harris AB (1997) Pediatric nutrition assessment: identifying children at risk. *Journal of the American Dietetic Association*. **97**(suppl 2): S107–S115.

Balen R, Fielding D and Lewis IJ (1998) An activity week for children with cancer: who wants to go and why? *Child: Care, Health and Development*. **24**: 169–77.

Bradford R (1997) *Children, Families and Chronic Disease*. Routledge, London.

Budd KS, McGraw TE, Farbisz R, Murphy TB, Hawkins D, Heilman N, Werle M and Hochstadt NJ (1992) Psychosocial concomitants of children's feeding disorders. *Journal of Pediatric Psychology*. **17**: 81–94.

Cairns GF and Altman K (1979) Behavioral treatment of cancer-related anorexia. *Journal of Behavior Therapy and Experimental Psychiatry*. **10**: 353–6.

Carey S (1985) *Conceptual Change in Childhood*. MIT Press, Massachusetts.

Culbert AP, Kajander RL, Kohen DP and Reaney JB (1996) Hypnobehavioral approaches for school-age children with dysphagia and food aversion: a case series. *Developmental and Behavioral Pediatrics*. **17**: 335–41.

Dale N (1996) *Working with Families of Children with Special Needs*. Routledge, London.

Douglas J (1995) Behavioural eating disorders in young children. *Current Paediatrics*. **5**: 39–42.

Douglas J, Hulson B and Trompeter RS (1998) Psycho-social outcome of parents and young children after renal transplantation. *Child: Care, Health and Development*. **24**: 73–83.

Drotar D (1997) Intervention research: pushing back the frontiers of pediatric psychology. *Journal of Pediatric Psychology*. **22**: 593–606.

Eiser C (1990) *Childhood Chronic Disease*. Cambridge University Press, Cambridge.

Eiser C (1998) Long term consequences of childhood cancer. *Journal of Child Psychology and Psychiatry*. **39**: 621–33.

Elander J and Midence K (1997) Children with chronic illness. *The Psychologist*. March: 1–5.

Epston D (1994) Strange and novel ways of addressing guilt. In: D Epston and M White (eds) *Experience, Contradiction, Narrative and Imagination*. Dulwich Centre Publications, Adelaide.

Erikson E (1980) *Identity and the Life Cycle*. Norton, New York.

Evans J and le Grange D (1995) Body side and parenting in eating disorders: a comparative study of the attitudes of mothers towards their children. *International Journal of Eating Disorders*. **18**(1): 39–48.

Fielding D (1985) Chronic illness in children. In: FN Watts (ed) *New Developments in Clinical Psychology*. British Psychological Society Books, Leicester.

Hellin K and Waller G (1992) Mothers' mood and infant feeding: prediction of problems and practices. *Journal of Reproductive and Infant Psychology*. **10**: 39–51.

Hoch TA, Babbitt RL, Coe DA, Krell DM and Hackbert L (1994) Contingency contracting. *Behavior Modification*. **18**: 106–28.

Kelly GA (1955) *The Psychology of Personal Constructs*. Norton, New York.

Kelly K (1986) An overview of how to nourish the cancer patient by mouth. *Cancer*. **58**: 1897–1901.

Kendall PC and Norton-Ford JD (1982) *Clinical Psychology: scientific and professional dimensions*. Wiley and Sons, New York.

Kerwin ME and Berkowitz RI (1996) Feeding and eating disorders: ingestive problems of infancy, childhood and adolescence. *School Psychology Review*. **25**: 316–28.

Knafl K, Breitmeyer B, Gallo A and Zoeller L (1992) Parents' views of healthcare providers: an exploration of the components of a positive working relationship. *Child Health Care*. **21**: 90–5.

La Greca AM and Varni JW (1993) Editorial: Interventions in pediatric psychology: a look to the future. *Journal of Pediatric Psychology*. **18**: 667–79.

Leung AK and Robson WL (1994) The toddler who does not eat. *American Family Physician*. **49**: 1789–1800.

Linscheid TR (1998) Behavioral treatment of feeding disorders in children. In: TS Watson and FM Gresham (eds) *Handbook of Child Behavior Therapy*. Plenum Press, New York.

MacDonald A (1996) Nutritional management of cystic fibrosis. *Archives of Diseases in Childhood*. **74**: 81–7.

Melvin D, Wright C and Goddard S (1997) Incidence and nature of feeding problems in young children referred to a paediatric HIV service in London: FEAD screening. *Child: Care, Health and Development*. **23**(4): 297–313.

Neumark-Sztainer D, Story M, Toporoff E, Cassuto N, Resnick MD and Blum RW (1996) Psychosocial predictors of binge eating and purging behaviours among adolescents with and without diabetes mellitus. *Journal of Adolescent Health*. **19**: 289–96.

O'Brien S, Repp AC, Williams GE and Christophersen ER (1991) Pediatric feeding disorders. *Behavior Modification*. **15**: 394–418.

Padilla GV and Grant MM (1985) Psychosocial aspects of artificial feeding. *Cancer*. **55**: 301–4.

Pearson DA, Pumariega AJ and Seilheimer DK (1991) The development of psychiatric symptomatology in patients with cystic fibrosis. *Journal of the American Academy of Child and Adolescent Psychiatry.* **30**: 290–7.

Piaget J (1976) *Six Psychological Studies.* New York, Vintage Books.

Pless IB and Roghmann KJ (1971) Chronic illness and its consequences: observations based on three epidemiologic surveys. *Journal of Pediatrics.* **79**: 351–9.

Pollock M, Kovacs M and Charron-Prochownik D (1995) Eating disorders and maladaptive dietary/insulin management among youths with childhood onset insulin dependent diabetes mellitus. *Journal of the American Academy of Child and Adolescent Psychiatry.* **34**: 291–6.

Ravelli AM (1995) Gasrointestinal function in chronic renal failure. *Pediatric Nephrology.* **9**: 756–62.

Rickhard KA, Coates TD, Grosfield JL, Weetman RM and Baehner RL (1986) The value of nutrition support in children with cancer. *Cancer.* **58**: 1904–10.

Ross DM and Ross SA (1988) *Childhood Pain.* Urban & Schwarzenberg, Baltimore.

Russell GFM, Treasure J and Eisler I (1998) Mothers with anorexia nervosa who underfeed their children: their recognition and management. *Psychological Medicine.* **28**: 93–108.

Sadowski RH, Allred EN and Jabs K (1993) Sodium modelling ameliorates intradialytic and interdialytic symptoms in young haemodialysis patients. *Journal of the American Society of Nephrology.* **4**: 1192–8.

Sanders MR, Turner KMT, Wall CR, Waugh LM and Tully LA (1997) Mealtime behavior and parent–child interaction: a comparison of children with cystic fibrosis, children with feeding problems, and nonclinic controls. *Journal of Pediatric Psychology.* **22**: 881–900.

Schwartz AL (1997) *Relationship Dimensions in Treatment Adherence: the use of repertory grids.* European Psychosocial Working Group for Children with Chronic Renal Failure, Lille.

Schwartz AL and Mercer A (1998) The role of the clinical psychologist in paediatric pain management. In: A Twycross, A Moriarty and T Betts (eds) *Paediatric Pain Management: a multidisciplinary approach.* Radcliffe Medical Press, Oxford.

Shepherd M, Oppenheim B and Mitchell S (1971) *Childhood Behavior and Mental Health.* University of London Press, London.

Singer LT, Nofer JA, Benson-Szekely LJ and Brooks LJ (1991) Behavioral assessment and management of food refusal in children with cystic fibrosis. *Developmental and Behavioral Pediatrics.* **12**: 115–19.

Sokel B, Devane S, Bentovim A and Milla PJ (1991) Self hypnotherapeutic treatment of habitual reflex vomiting. *Archives of Diseases in Childhood.* **65**: 626–7.

Stein A, Stein J, Walters EA and Fairburn CG (1995) Eating attitudes among mothers of children with feeding disorders. *British Medical Journal.* **310**: 228.

Strologo LD, Principato F, Sinibaldi D, Appiani AC, Terzi F, Dartois AE and Rizzoni G

(1997) Feeding dysfunction in infants with severe chronic renal failure after long-term nasogastric tubefeeding. *Pediatric Nephrology*. **11**: 84–6.

Tawfik R, Dickson A, Clarke M and Thomas AG (1997) Caregivers' perceptions following gastrostomy in severely disabled children with feeding problems. *Developmental Medicine and Child Neurology*. **39**: 746–51.

van Eys J (1979) Malnutrition in children with cancer. *Cancer*. **43**: 2030–5.

Warady BA, Kriley M, Belden B, Hellerstein S and Alun U (1990) Nutritional and behavioural aspects of nasogastric tube-feeding in infants receiving chronic peritoneal dialysis. *Advances in Peritoneal Dialysis*. **6**: 265–8.

Wardley BL, Puntis JWL and Taitz LS (1997) *Handbook of Child Nutrition*. Oxford University Press, Oxford.

Werle MA, Murphy TB and Budd KS (1993) Treating chronic food refusal in young children: home based parent training. *Journal of Applied Behavioral Analysis*. **26**: 421–33.

WHO (1992) *The ICD-10 Classification of Mental and Behavioural Disorders: clinical descriptions and diagnostic guidelines*. World Health Organisation, Geneva.

Woody RC (1990) The role of the pediatric neurologist in feeding disorders. *Journal of Neurological Rehabilitation*. **4**: 97–101.

Wooster DM, Brady NR, Mitchell A, Grizzle MH and Barnes M (1998) Pediatric feeding: a transdisciplinary team's perspective. *Topics in Language Disorders*. **18**: 34–51.

Zeltzer LK, Dolgin MJ, Sahler OJ, Roghman K, Barbarin OA, Carpenter PJ, Copeland DR, Mulhern RK and Sargent JR (1996) Sibling adaptation to childhood cancer collaborative study: health outcomes of siblings of children with cancer. *Medical Pediatric Oncology*. **27**: 98–107.

Further reading

Altschuler J (1997) *Working with Chronic Illness*. Macmillan Press, London.

American Psychiatric Association (1994) *Diagnostic and Statistical Manual of Mental Disorders (4e)*. American Psychiatric Association, Washington DC.

Anderson CA and Lock J (1997) Feeding disorders. In: H Steiner (ed) *Treating Pre-School Children*. Jossey-Bass Publishers, San Francisco.

Black MM and Teti LO (1997) Promoting mealtime communication between adolescent mothers and their infants through videotape. *Pediatrics*. **99**: 432–7.

Briggs S (1997) *Growth and Risk in Infancy*. Jessica Kingsley, London.

Callum R, Waller G, Cox A and Slade A (1997) Eating attitudes in young teenage girls: parental management of 'fussy' eating. *Eating Disorders*. **5**: 29–40.

Daws D (1993) Feeding problems and relationship difficulties: therapeutic work with parents and infants. *Journal of Child Psychotherapy*. **19**: 69–84.

Daws D (1997) The perils of intimacy: closeness and distance in feeding and weaning. *Journal of Child Psychotherapy.* **23**: 179–93.

Drotar D (1994) Coming of age: critical challenges to the future development of pediatric psychology. *Journal of Pediatric Psychology.* **16**: 1–11.

Engel GL (1977) The need for a new medical model: challenge for biomedicine. *Science.* **196**: 129–36.

Engel GL (1980) The clinical application of the biopsychosocial model. *American Journal of Psychiatry.* **137**: 535–44.

Holaday M, Smith KE, Robertson S and Dallas J (1994) An atypical eating disorder with Crohn's disease in a fifteen year old male: a case study. *Adolescence.* **29**: 865–73.

Lavigne JV and Faier-Routman J (1992) Psychological adjustment to pediatric physical disorders: a meta-analytic review. *Journal of Pediatric Psychology.* **17**: 133–57.

Lindberg L, Bohlin G and Hagekull B (1991) Early feeding problems in a normal population. *International Journal of Eating Disorders.* **10**: 395–405.

Lindscheid TR (1992) Eating problems in children. In: CE Walker and MC Roberts (eds) *Handbook of Clinical Child Psychology.* Wiley and Sons, New York.

NHS Health Advisory Service (1995) *Review of Child and Adolescent Mental Health Services: together we stand.* Department of Health, London.

NHS Management Advisory Service (1989) *National Review of Clinical Psychology Services.* National Health Service, London.

Parry A and Doan RE (1994) *Story Revisions: narrative therapy in the post-modern world.* Guilford Press, New York.

Reimers S and Street E (1993) Using family therapy in child and adolescent services. In: J Carpenter and A Treacher (eds) *Using Family Therapy in the Nineties.* Blackwell, Oxford.

Richman N, Stevenson J and Graham PJ (1992) *Pre-school to School: a behavioural study.* Academic Press, London.

Roberts MC (1986) *Pediatric Psychology.* Pergamon Press, New York.

Singer L and Drotar D (1989) Psychological practice in a paediatric rehabilitation hospital. *Journal of Pediatric Psychology.* **14**: 479–89.

Skuse D, Wolke D and Reilly S (1992) Failure to thrive: clinical and developmental aspects. In: H Reschmidt and MH Schmidt (eds) *Developmental Psychopathology.* Hofgrefe and Huber, New York.

Spence SH (1994) Practitioner review: cognitive therapy with children and adolescents: from theory to practice. *Journal of Child Psychology and Psychiatry.* **35**: 1191–228.

Stein A and Fairburn CG (1994) An infant with cystic fibrosis and a mother with an eating disorder: a difficult combination. *International Journal of Eating Disorders.* **16**(1): 93–5.

Wallander JL (1992) Theory driven research in pediatric psychology: a little bit on why and how. *Journal of Pediatric Psychology.* **17**: 521–35.

CHAPTER 14

Cross-cultural understanding and the management of feeding problems

Pratibha Rao

Introduction

The traditional definition of culture is the customs and civilisations of a particular group of people. Culture influences virtually all aspects of human behaviour and practices and perhaps none more so than food and feeding habits.

Ethnic minority groups feature in the populations of a number of European and American societies. This chapter is concerned with the UK, with a particular focus on Asian populations. It cannot hope to be definitive in its discussions of such a wide-ranging, multifaceted topic. It is hoped, however, that it may give the reader something of an insight into the special considerations necessary when working with families of ethnic minority origin, or whose family culture is different from their own.

Epidemiological factors

Ethnic minorities make up around 6% of the total population of the UK. The largest group of these originate from India, followed by those of African-Caribbean and Pakistani origin. Also, very importantly, an ever-increasing proportion of the ethnic minorities are British-born, making them an overall younger population. It follows that children constitute a significantly higher percentage of the total, as compared to the indigenous UK population. Thus, health-related issues that pertain to young, ethnic minority individuals, and their nutritional status in particular, are important issues which need to be specifically addressed when formulating health policy.

Social and family issues

A disproportionate number of ethnic minority children come from disadvantaged families concentrated in inner city areas where there is high unemployment and overcrowding. In Asian households, two-parent families are generally the norm and single motherhood relatively uncommon. Also the elders, especially mothers-in-law, exercise a great deal of influence over the diet of children. In the author's experience, Asian elders generally worry a great deal about food intake of youngsters, many believing that being plump is a sign of good health. Many first-generation Asians may have language and communication difficulties which do not apply to the second generation born and bred in Britain. However, Asian children growing up in the UK face difficulties trying to balance traditional values and practices taught at home with the vastly different 'Westernised' norms and beliefs they imbibe at school and from the world outside. Acculturation is an important aspect of ethnicity and refers to the extent to which an individual's cultural beliefs change as a result of influences from the mainstream culture. It follows that acculturation greatly affects diet and feeding practices within families.

In black households, too, there is a high rate of unemployment and black households are far more likely to become statutorally homeless than white (Association of Metropolitan Authorities 1990). Also African-Caribbean children are more likely to be taken into local authority care than Asian or white children. In general, a high proportion of ethnic minority families in the UK suffer poverty and disadvantage, both of which exert a detrimental effect on the diet and nutrition of children within these families.

Religious issues

Religion plays a very important role in influencing dietary practices of many ethnic groups. Hindus do not generally eat beef; Muslims shun pork and usually consume 'Halal' meat. Vegetarianism is particularly prevalent in the Gujarati Hindu community in the UK. Families of African-Caribbean background tend to be predominantly Christian, with no particular religious influences on their diet. The exception is the Rastafarian sect, a small minority of African-Caribbean people who are vegetarian. Generally speaking, the traditional foods eaten by these various ethnic groups are more nutritious than the typical Western diet, which is made up of more refined foods. However, there are significant medical problems relating to certain vitamin and nutrient deficiencies resulting from vegetarian and vegan diets and these are discussed later.

Age-specific feeding problems in relation to culture – the neonatal period

Breast-feeding

Of all aspects of infant feeding, perhaps none is more strongly influenced by culture and ethnicity than breast-feeding. A substantial number of studies have been performed recently in the USA and UK, as well as parts of the developed world, looking at breast-feeding practices in various communities. Overall in the UK breast-feeding rates have increased in the past 20 years. Initial breast-feeding rates in 1995 were 68% in England and Wales, 55% in Scotland and 45% in Northern Ireland (Foster *et al.* 1997). A Department of Health survey carried out in England (Thomas and Avery 1997) showed a significantly higher incidence of breast-feeding among Asian mothers as compared to white mothers living in the same areas. The figures quoted are 62% among white mothers, 92% among Bangladeshis, 82% among Indians and 76% for Pakistani mothers. Despite higher rates of initial breast-feeding, the survey showed that by eight weeks the levels had declined in all four groups. In addition, Asian mothers, particularly those of Bangladeshi origin, are more likely to give their babies top-up feeds because of worries of insufficient milk. In the parent countries, too (in particular India and Pakistan), there has been recent widespread media concern over the overall decline in breast-feeding rates secondary to advertising by milk companies and also a rise in the population of middle-class, working mothers.

Acculturation is an important determinant of breast-feeding. Various studies of immigrant populations have found that acculturation exerts a negative effect on breast-feeding, namely, that the more 'Westernised' mothers become, the less likely they are to breast-feed than their traditional counterparts (Rassim *et al.* 1993, 1994).

While in white mothers in the UK maternal age, level of education and social class are important determinants of breast-feeding, such correlations in Asian women are far less clear cut (Thomas and Avery 1997). This may, of course, be partly a result of the social disadvantages already mentioned, which confound education and social class variables. It is interesting that in the African and African-Caribbean populations, breast-feeding rates are high both within the UK and in the countries of origin (Ineichen 1995). In this group, acculturation has had no significant impact on breast-feeding.

Practicalities of breast-feeding

Asian mothers frequently report sickness or sore nipples as reasons for not breast-feeding (Evans *et al.* 1976). Insufficient milk supply is another common reason for termination of breast-feeding (Thomas and Avery 1997). However, a study in Illinois concluded that insufficient milk supply was not related to ethnicity and found that the incidence of reduced milk supply was similar for black and white mothers (Hill and Aldag 1993).

A widespread belief among Asian elders is that colostrum is harmful for babies. Some Asian women prefer not to feed their babies colostrum but to wait until the mature milk is through. The recent infant feeding survey in England showed that a significant number of Asian mothers delay breast-feeding until they get home, although very few mention a fear of colostrum as the reason for this (Thomas and Avery 1997).

The interpretations of breast-feeding difficulties are illustrated by the following case example.

> *Case example 1: A three-month-old Asian boy was referred to the outpatients department of a busy inner city hospital with stridor (i.e. noise on inspiration). He was born by normal delivery at term in Pakistan with a birth weight of 3.2 kg. Mother was born and bred in Pakistan. She was a devoted Muslim and wore a veil. She had been married at the age of 18 to a Pakistani settled in Britain. When she became pregnant she returned to Pakistan to have her baby. She received no antenatal care in England. She came back to Britain to rejoin her husband when the baby was a month old. The child was breast-fed and thriving. However, he was described as being some-what erratic with feeds. His breathing was noted to be extremely noisy from the age of about 3–4 weeks. The paternal grandmother who lived with the couple in England was convinced that faulty breast milk was the cause of the problem.*

On initial assessment the child appeared well. Weight and head circumferences were on the 10th centile in keeping with birth measurements. There was mild stridor but no recession. There was a degree of craniotabes but no other signs of rickets. Initial investigations revealed a low serum calcium of 1.2 mmol/l. This was repeated several times and found to be consistently low. Subsequently vitamin D levels in both mother and baby were found to be low. Alkaline phosphatase was moderately high. The baby was treated initially with calcium supplements for a fortnight. He was also put on One-Alpha (alfacalcidol), which was continued for six weeks and thereafter he was put on standard baby vitamin supplementation. The mother also was given vitamin D. The baby's symptoms, i.e. stridor, settled rapidly thereafter and serum calcium returned to normal within a few weeks. When seen six months later the infant was very well and was discharged from further follow-up. He was still breast-fed and was also receiving a weaning diet. There was no further conflict between the child's mother and the elders within the extended family. It would appear that, in this instance, there had been a matching of the medical intervention with the belief system of the family (*see* Chapter 6 for a further discussion of professional–parent relationships regarding feeding problems).

Strategies to improve breast-feeding

Several studies have demonstrated that educating mothers about the beneficial effects of breast-feeding in the prenatal period may be highly effective (Timbo *et al.* 1996). Encouragement by physicians is also reportedly an important factor in influencing women. The author's experience with Asian mothers with pre-term babies suggests that virtually all of them respond to doctors' advice on the benefits of breast milk for their premature baby.

- Health visitors and midwives need to be aware of and sensitive to the cultural influences of breast-feeding when advising young mothers.
- Breast-feeding issues need to be discussed antenatally.
- Where there are language and communication difficulties between health professionals and women, interpreters may be invaluable. One hopes that with the increasing number of doctors, nurses and various other healthcare professionals in the NHS who are, themselves, of ethnic minority origin, such communication difficulties may be overcome. At all times professionals need to maintain a caring, sympathetic and non-patronising attitude.

Weaning diet

The reader is referred to a detailed review on this subject by James and Underwood (1997). Weaning refers to the introduction of solid and liquid food other than milk (breast or formula) to an infant. Weaning is important not only to fulfil the nutritional needs of the child, but also to enable the child to experience new tastes and different consistencies of food. Thereby the infant gradually learns to chew and swallow. It is generally recommended that solids are introduced at around four months and lumpy foods by 6–7 months, aiming for the child to be on a regular mixed diet and able to partake of a family meal by the age of one year. In general, weaning occurs later in Asian and Chinese populations. In addition, Asian children tend to drink inappropriate volumes of cow's milk for a long time at the expense of solid food. Asian children also tend to use feeding bottles for a longer time, occasionally up to and beyond school age. In developing countries, too, the problems of increased malnutrition in association with delayed weaning have been highlighted (Chirmulay and Nisal 1993).

Types of weaning foods

Again these vary enormously and are determined not just by ethnicity but also by income and social class. Vegetarian foods are commonly used among the Indian population and vegan diets may be practised among Rastafarians.

The Department of Health survey on infant feeding revealed that 24% of Indian households were vegetarian. At nine months 38% of Indian children never ate meat, while nearly all Bengali, Pakistani and white households ate meat. Asian babies took longer than white babies to establish a mixed diet and Bangladeshi babies in particular ate a narrower range of foods than white children.

Feeding behaviour

At 15 months white children are more likely than Asian children to feed themselves. White, Indian and Pakistani children were more likely to drink from a cup or beaker than Bangladeshi children. Asian mothers tend to worry a lot about their child's food intake. Bangladeshi mothers were more likely to say their child had a poor appetite, was fussy or difficult to feed and white mothers were least likely to voice such concerns (Thomas and Avery 1997).

Growth-related issues in infancy

The results of the infant feeding survey in England suggest that birth weight on average is higher for white than Asian infants. At nine weeks white babies were heavier than Asian babies; at 15 months white boys were heavier than Asian boys. However, Pakistani and Indian girls of this age were of similar weight to white girls but Bangladeshi girls were lighter. White boys and girls had a larger head circumference at all ages than Asian infants.

The three main factors associated with weight at 15 months in all groups were birth weight, sex and parental height. Asian children were also likely to be lighter if their mothers reported persistent feeding problems, i.e. not eating enough/not interested in food (Thomas and Avery 1997).

Supine length at 15 months appears to be related to length at nine weeks, parental height and sex (girls were likely to be shorter than boys in all groups except Indian). Also Indian children given cow's milk at nine months tended to be taller.

Growth monitoring in ethnic minority children

The recommendation of the Hall Report is that standard growth foundation charts be used for all children in Britain including those from ethnic minorities. While it is recognised that African-Caribbean children tend to be slightly taller than Asian children and slightly smaller than white Caucasian children, these differences probably reflect parental heights rather than ethnic origin.

Issues surrounding the management of a child with failure to thrive are emphasised by the following example of clinical practice. The factors relating to family structure, gender and therapeutic approach highlight the need to maintain cultural awareness.

> *Case example 2: A seven-year-old girl of Bangladesh origin was being followed up in paediatric clinic for food refusal and failure to thrive. She was born normally at 38 weeks gestation with a birth weight of 2.6 kg. Birth and development was normal. She was bottle-fed and described as a poor feeder from early infancy, taking a long time to complete her bottles. Her weight gain in the early months was somewhat suboptimal and she was therefore changed on to Wysoy with a presumed diagnosis of cow's milk intolerance. At around four months she was also weaned on to jars of baby food. At the age of six months she went with her parents to Bangladesh and spent the next 18 months there. While in Bangladesh she developed chronic diarrhoea with a further tailing off of weight. When her symptoms improved she was put on to cow's milk and a traditional Asian diet including lentils, rice and fish, etc., but she remained very difficult to feed. At the age of two she returned to the UK.*
>
> *Family history: Her father was in his late twenties, a chef by profession who owned his own restaurant. Her mother, who was a couple of years younger, did not work outside the home. Both sets of grandparents lived in the UK but not within daily commuting distance. The family were devoted Muslims.*
>
> *During pre-school and early school years, the child was under close surveillance by the health visitor and GP but her growth*

remained just above the 3rd centile and she was therefore never referred to hospital. At the age of seven years she was admitted with a 'funny turn', felt to be a fit. All investigations at that stage, including an electroencephalogram (EEG), were normal. Her parents admitted to hospital staff that they were very concerned about her behaviour. Indeed this had been a long-standing problem. From being an awkward feeder as an infant she had progressed to being a rather difficult toddler and her negative behaviour had continued right up to the present time. She was described as 'naughty and disobedient and always quarrelling with mother'. There appeared to be some worsening of her behaviour following the birth of her brother who was three years younger than herself. The main problem was food refusal. The child seemed to dislike eating in general and refused to take anything that had as much as a hint of spice in it. She generally tended to misbehave for her mother. Her father, however, did exercise some control over her and would often, by cajoling and threatening, manage to get her to eat small amounts at meal times. There was no significant vomiting and her bowels were normal.

Following her hospital admission, her behaviour in general and food refusal in particular got significantly worse. She was seen in clinic six months later and at that point had lost 3.5 kg in weight, drifting from the 10th to below the 3rd centile, and her parents said she was stubborn and uncommunicative. She would eat very little (both at home and at school) and took a long time to complete even a small amount. She never seemed hungry. Her mother appreciated her dislike of spicy foods at home and completely changed the diet to make it more palatable to the child. She tried offering her plain lentils and rice and even small amounts of English food, but to no avail. She sent a packed lunch to school, mostly sandwiches and these, too, were returned home largely untouched. A dietician's assessment during this period was that the food was entirely satisfactory in quality but certainly not in quantity. The child's behaviour during this time remained as difficult as ever. She was rude and quarrelsome to her mother. She was also rather disruptive in school and it was becoming clear that she had some learning difficulties.

At this point she was referred to the child and adolescent psychiatrist, who undertook a comprehensive assessment together with a team of nurses trained in the management of behaviour problems in children. As a result of the assessment it immediately became clear that the child's hospital admission six months previously had worsened an already precarious situation. The child, who was naturally stubborn and wilful, had realised that refusing food was causing her parents a great deal of consternation and seemed to be using this to her advantage. The father's rather domineering and inflexible attitude was not helpful. The child was invited to attend the ward for further assessment. While she was there she integrated very well with the other children. She was offered a standard English meal of fish, chips and vegetables. Once her parents were out of sight the child ate her meal without any fuss.

The staff drew up a careful management strategy. Apart from the child's weekly attendance, the parents were invited to attend monthly meetings. At these sessions parental attitudes to their children in general, and their daughter's eating behaviour in particular, were explored at length and some interesting observations were made.

- The father was somewhat dismissive of the female members of the team but was far more attentive to the males, therefore a male member (a consultant psychiatrist) was specifically assigned to chair these sessions.
- Both parents were asked to air their views individually thus allowing the child's normally reticent mother to be heard.
- The mother's attitude to the child was essentially sympathetic and tolerant. Furthermore, she treated both children similarly. The father, on the other hand, was agitated and annoyed by his daughter's behaviour and was far more accepting of his son's behaviour (also rather mischievous and attention-seeking) as that of a 'normal' toddler.

Following on from the initial assessment of family dynamics, the parents were counselled at length. The father was advised to stop being too dictatorial about the child's food. The mother was advised to (a) give her daughter the usual family meals but without including spices and (b) encourage her to eat as much as she could but not get perturbed if she didn't complete the meal and just clear up afterwards with no comment. Meanwhile the child continued to attend for weekly assessment. Over the next 3–4 months there was a rapid improvement in her feeding habits. It appeared as though the very process of being allowed some freedom at meal times without the constant pressure of being watched and coaxed into eating more, seemed to make meal times less of an ordeal and more pleasurable. There was a marked improvement in her eating behaviours and although she continued to have the odd day when she would misbehave, she did, on the whole, start to eat much better. She regained virtually all the weight she had lost within a few months. At the time of writing, she continues to undergo assessment and is likely to be discharged provided her progress remains good.

Food-related issues in older children

Ethnic minority children of school age in the UK tend to eat a combination of traditional food cooked at home and standard 'English' fare consumed by their white classmates. In general, parental education and parental income seem to be more important determinants of a nutritious diet in school children than ethnic origin alone.

Whereas most traditional foods tend to be high in fibre, some studies have found high fat and salt contents, particularly in the diets of African-Caribbean origin (Nicklas *et al.* 1995). Some specific nutritional problems related to ethnicity are given in Box 14.1.

Box 14.1: Specific medical/nutritional problems related to ethnicity

- Vitamin D deficiency: Asian children are particularly at risk from infancy through to late childhood. The following reasons may contribute:
  - vitamin D-deficient mothers produce vitamin D-deficient breast milk – hypocalcaemia and its effects, biochemical and florid rickets are all recognised in Asian infants
  - weaning diets may be lacking in vitamin D
  - poverty is an important factor associated with rickets
  - shielding the skin from sunlight may be a factor in some rachitic children.
- Iron-deficiency anaemia: children of Asian and Afro-Caribbean origin in the UK appear to have a greater incidence of iron deficiency than their white counterparts. This may rather be the result of poverty than ethnicity alone. Risk factors for the development of iron-deficiency anaemia, especially in Asian children, include:
  - excess of cow's milk in the first year of life
  - late weaning
  - weaning on to vegetarian diets which are low in iron
  - lack of breast-feeding.

Prevention of iron-deficiency anaemia

All primary health workers need to be aware of the problem and to give appropriate dietary advice. The use of iron-fortified formulae has been shown to reduce the incidence of iron-deficiency anaemia, although the practicalities/ costs of using such formulae need to be explored. Iron supplementation is, of course, recommended, when the diagnosis is made. However, routine screening for iron-deficiency anaemia is not recommended at the present time (Hall Report 1996).

Obesity

The incidence of obesity may vary according to ethnicity, with some studies finding that children from some black and East-Asian subgroups tend to be more obese than their white peers. Studies suggest that dietary habits are responsible and that dietary modification can be a successful intervention (McNutt *et al.* 1997; Ray and Lim 1994). It seems likely, however, that for some groups the 'culture of thinness', which has become so predominant in European and American cultures, has yet to fully permeate. For example, in the Asian community, thin children are usually the source of much anxiety among elders and overweight children are often perceived as 'healthy'. Although thinness has not traditionally been seen as a desirable quality in black and Asian populations, the rising incidence of eating disorders such as anorexia and bulimia nervosa among ethnic minorities in Britain suggests that this may be changing (Mumford *et al.* 1991).

Summary

In today's multiethnic Britain, many families from ethnic minorities suffer poverty and social disadvantage, which adversely affect the nutritional status of their young. Initial breast-feeding rates are higher among black and Asian women than Caucasians but many mothers discontinue breast-feeding within a few months. Weaning generally occurs later, especially in Asian and Chinese populations. Specific medical problems that occur more frequently in ethnic minority children include iron-deficiency anaemia and vitamin D deficiency. Obesity and eating disorders such as anorexia are also being increasingly recognised. In this chapter it has been shown that culture and ethnicity exert a powerful influence on dietary practices within a community. The role of acculturation has been touched on, as well as the importance of understanding the traditional beliefs about food. These issues serve as an important backdrop to situations where feeding problems occur. There is now an increasing awareness among health professionals of the cultural, social and health issues that pertain to ethnic minority children. It is hoped that in the years to come their nutritional status and consequently their physical and emotional health will continue to improve.

References

Association of Metropolitan Authorities (1990) *Report of Local Authority Housing and Racial Equality Working Party*. HMSO, London.

Chirmulay D and Nisal R (1993) Nutritional status of tribal under 5 children in Ahmadnagar District, Maharashtra in relation to weaning/feeding practices. *Indian Paediatrics*. **30**(2): 215–22.

Evans N, Walpole IR, Qureshi MU, Menon HM, Everly Jones HW (1976) Lack of breast feeding in early weaning of infants of Asian immigrants in Wolverhampton. *Archives of Disease in Childhood*. **51**: 608–12.

Foster K, Cheesbrough S and Lader D (1997) *Infant Feeding 1995*. The Stationery Office, London.

Hall DMB (1996) *Health for All Children*. Oxford University Press, Oxford.

Hill PD and Aldag JC (1993) Insufficient milk supply among black and white breast-feeding mothers. *Research in Nursing and Health*. **16**(3): 203–11.

Ineichen B (1995) Strategies to promote breastfeeding in inner cities. *Health Visitor*. **68**(2): 61–2.

James J and Underwood A (1997) Ethnic influences on weaning diet in the UK. *Proceedings of the Nutrition Society*. **56**: 121–30.

McNutt SW, Hu Y, Schreiber GB, Crawford PB, Obarzanek E and Mellin L (1997) A longitudinal study of the dietary practices of black and white girls 9 and 10 years old at enrollment: the NHLBI Growth and Health Study. *Journal of Adolescent Health*. **20**(1): 27–37.

Mumford DB, Whitehouse AM and Platts M (1991) Sociocultural correlates of eating disorders among Asian schoolgirls in Bradford. *British Journal of Psychiatry*. **158**: 222–8.

Nicklas TA, Myers L and Berenson GS (1995) Dietary fiber intake of children: the Bogalusa Heart Study. *Paediatrics*. **96**(5 Pt 2): 988–94.

Rassim DK, Markides KS, Baranowski T, Mikrut WD, Winkler BA, Bee DE and Richardson CJ (1993) Acculturation and breast feeding on the United States-Mexico border. *American Journal of the Medical Sciences*. **306**(1): 28–34.

Rassim DK, Markides KS, Baranowski T, Richardson CJ, Mikrut WD and Bee DE (1994) Aculturation and the initiation of breast feeding. *Journal of Clinical Epidemiology*. **47**(7): 739–46.

Ray R and Lim LH (1994) Obesity in preschool children: an intervention programme in primary healthcare in Singapore. *Annals of the Academy of Medicine, Singapore*. **23**(3): 335–41.

Thomas M and Avery V (1997) *Infant feeding in Asian families*. A survey carried out in England by the Social Survey Division of ONS on behalf of the Department of Health. The Stationery Office, London.

Timbo B, Altekruse S and Headrick M (1996) Breastfeeding among black mothers: evidence supporting the need for prenatal intervention. *Journal of the Society of Paediatric Nurses*. **1**(1): 35–40.

CHAPTER 15

The feeding clinic

Sally Hodges and Rebecca Harris

Introduction

This chapter focuses on the development of a multidisciplinary, comprehensive treatment package for parents and their children with a feeding difficulty.

The literature on the management of feeding difficulties has tended to focus on treatment of specific aspects of the feeding process. The aspect that appears to receive the most input is that of the child's contribution to the difficulty, with treatment focusing on 'behavioural management' (Luiselli and Luiselli 1995; Luiselli 1994) or positioning and equipment (Griggs *et al.* 1989; Reilly and Skuse 1992; Gisel 1990), introducing a modified diet (Alexander 1987) or desensitisation (Alexander 1987). There is an enormous range of treatment literature with a child focus and a wide range of treatment recommendations from a large number of professional disciplines. A number of authors have focused on the adult (parental) factors, for example behavioural parent training, parent support groups (Chamberlin *et al.* 1991) or the parent–child relationship (Daws 1993). However, there are few examples in the literature of approaching the difficulties at more than one level simultaneously. There may be a number of reasons for this. First, therapists tend to be trained or have expertise in specific areas. There are obvious financial implications for widening the remit of treatment to a 'biopsychosocial' model, as it could create the need for a range of therapists who have the relevant background and skills. The biopsychosocial model, as described by Dale (1996), takes a multidimensional approach to causality and treatment, drawing on the biological, psychological and social aspects of the process of development of the child and family.

Second, working with disabled children can raise anxieties and uncomfortable feelings in staff, and the need to separate specific aspects of care to relieve the impact on the workers has been well documented (Menzies-Lyth 1988).

In this chapter, the process of setting up a feeding group programme for children with severe feeding difficulties and special needs is discussed. The programme consisted of two groups, one for parents and one for their children, and was designed to approach treatment from a number of levels, including the physical (biological), psychological and social. Issues, both practical and theoretical, arising through the process of setting up and running of the groups are explored.

The origins of the feeding group programme

Often children with developmental delay and feeding difficulties are receiving treatment concurrently from a number of different professionals. For instance, health visitors, community and specialist nurses are often involved, especially when the feeding difficulty had a physical origin or there are continued medical needs, such as a gastrostomy. Paediatricians, GPs, social workers, speech and language therapists, psychologists, occupational therapists and physiotherapists may all be involved in the treatment of the child's feeding difficulties. In some services, these workers may be providing a coordinated team approach. Indeed the 1989 Children Act specifically states that in all areas of childcare, including the area of children in need, professionals from different agencies should be working closely together.

Unfortunately, more often than not, services are disparate and unconnected, and there is often a haphazard or piecemeal approach to who receives what service or professional in their care package. The feeding group programme was set up partly in response to the identified service need of providing a coordinated approach to this client group and partly as a project with a clear theoretical basis, to address the different levels of causality and maintenance of the difficulty; the child aspects; the child–parent aspects; and the parental (adult) aspects as described above.

The group treatment of these children and families had its origins within a multidisciplinary child development team. The development followed a process that had roots in a wide range of areas, including a feeding problems audit, the collation of parents' views, and some 'pilot' pieces of individual work.

The local healthcare trust survey

An audit of the prevalence of paediatric feeding difficulties within the local community served by the trust was completed by the clinical psychology department (Neill and Irvine 1994). The impetus behind this audit was to clarify the numbers of children with moderate to severe feeding difficulties within the community, if these children were receiving professional input and, if so, from which professional groups.

In addition, this audit gathered a wide range of data in order to explore to what degree the traditional approach of a dichotomous definition of organic and psychological factors was dominant, as this obviously would have implications for referrals to different professional groups. Without any evidence, it seemed that this split (i.e. between physical and psychological explanations) was guiding the professional involvement and management of the children's difficulties. The aim was to gain evidence as to the validity of this widely held view.

The local audit was completed by all health visitors within the healthcare trust. It identified 63 children under five years of age with feeding difficulties severe enough to warrant a referral to a specialist professional. The audit confirmed that these children's difficulties were being conceptualised as exclusively organic in about 30%, exclusively psychological in about 40% and about 30% were defined as having a combination of difficulties. It was found that once a child had been assigned to one of these categories, any further difficulties they developed were also conceptualised in the same way. It was also found that the classification that each child had received was arbitrary depending on which professional had initially assessed the child.

Single case study pilot

The benefits of taking biopsychosocial factors into account when working with children with special needs have been well documented (Dale 1996). Yet the audit completed within the locality appeared to demonstrate that these children's difficulties were not being approached in a systematic and thorough way. This finding was borne out in the authors' experience: when the speech therapy and psychology waiting lists were compared, it was found that a number of children had been referred to each service independently, with no mention of the referral to the other agency. It was decided to join forces in working with several children, for the speech therapist and psychologist to work together to provide a more comprehensive approach. In one such case, a boy aged three who had severe developmental delay was selected. He had a nasogastric tube fitted following refusal to take food orally as a consequence of a choking incident at one year. The child's parents were seen by the clinical psychologist, while the boy followed a desensitisation programme with the speech and language therapist. After four months of this approach oral feeding was reintroduced and the parents were able to continue this work at home with support visits from one of the group workers that started at once weekly and reduced over time.

Parents' views

A sample of parents' views was collected from parents who had been seen by the speech therapist, the psychologist and in the joint 'pilot'. The views of parents were also sought from the families of children on the waiting lists for feeding difficulties. Several important themes emerged from these views including:

- parents feeling isolated with their child's feeding difficulties
- confusion about the input from different professionals and misunderstandings arising from these
- some parents had previously attended feeding programmes in other centres, but had concerns about the distance they had to take their child, the amount of school missed and how these programmes were perceived as large, impersonal and not tailored to their child's needs.

It appeared that on the whole, the parents consulted were positive about the possibility of local, group-based treatment for their child's feeding difficulties.

The first feeding group programme

It was decided that group treatment was the most appropriate for a number of reasons:

- it was cost effective, given the apparent large numbers of children with feeding difficulties in the area
- there had been specific requests by the parents for group work
- group work has been indicated as successful with this client group (Chamberlin *et al.* 1991)
- the social support element provided by groups is important for caregivers dealing with feeding difficulties (Rosenthal *et al.* 1995).

Once the viability of the multidisciplinary approach had been established, a pilot group programme was developed. It was decided that as the group was a new venture, initially the group would be offered to a small number of families for a limited time period. Chamberlin *et al.* (1991) have described a similar support group for parents of children with special needs and feeding difficulties. The group they set up aimed to provide support, education and specific intervention strategies for the parents. This group also involved inviting outside professionals to give specific teaching input to the group. The group met with the children present, but it is not clear how this was organised or how the children's treatment was conducted within this group. Chamberlin *et al.* identified improvements in all six of the children seen in the range of foods accepted orally or quantity of foods accepted orally, or both areas. They described positive feedback from the parents they worked with, and concluded that group treatment could be a 'successful approach'. On the basis of the feedback from the pilot group, the ongoing group programme was established.

Selection criteria

In considering the selection criteria, it was recognised that a number of children often go through periods of food refusal or faddiness during the early years of development. However, the aim was to target those children who were demonstrating a serious or chronic feeding difficulty. The criteria that were finally agreed are given in Box 15.1.

Box 15.1: Criteria for acceptance into the group

- The child had identified special needs in more than one area of development
- The child was between 12 months and five years old
- The child had already received input from more than one other health professional around feeding
- The child had a history of medical intervention
- The child had severe feeding difficulties, with no ongoing medical cause
- The child had less severe, but chronic feeding difficulties
- The child was not expected to have any invasive medical treatment within the next six months

---

Initial assessments

Each family was invited to a pre-group meeting with the clinical psychologist and the speech therapist. The meeting involved taking a detailed developmental and medical history of the child, exploration of previous interventions and exploration of family issues around feeding. In addition, records of the family meal-time behaviour and the child's current intake of food (tube, oral or both) were obtained.

It was considered extremely important to clarify the expectations before the start of the group as, according to Wolf and Glass (1992), the parents or carers need to be ready to undertake a programme focused on oral feeding. Support in completing homework tasks outside of therapy sessions is also extremely important.

For this reason, an explanation of the aims of the programme was given to the family at this meeting, as well as the expectations of them, such as committing themselves to attending the group once a week for eight weeks, and completing tasks between sessions and during sessions. Where applicable, both parents were invited to the group, though it was asked that at least one of the parents attended consistently.

Staffing

In order to meet the needs of the children within the feeding group a high degree of support was required, often on a one-to-one basis. At all times the children's group was staffed by four adults to six children. The staff were drawn from the speech therapy department, a play specialist was employed for the duration of the group and other staff volunteered to assist at various points. These included the pre-school home visitor (portage) workers attached to each child, students on placement with either the speech therapy or psychology departments and specialist health visitors. Before the start of each session, all the staff involved met to plan the session and to discuss relevant issues that had arisen from the previous groups. Box 15.2 outlines a plan for the session.

Box 15.2: The feeding group timetable

12.00–12.30	Pre-group professionals meeting to discuss plans for the group
12.30–12.40	Groups start together; parents settle children in
12.40–1.40	Groups meet separately
1.00–1.30	Where a guest speaker has been organised, they attend at this time
1.40ish	Parents and children's groups join together for feedback
1.50	Clear up followed by professionals debrief meeting

Practical considerations

The children's group took place in a large room within the child development centre. The room contained sinks and was next door to a kitchen, with easy access to a fridge, freezer and microwave. The adults met in an adjacent room that was separated from the children's group room by dividing doors. The group met on a weekly basis, at lunch time, to enable the children to experience food associated with a typical meal time. Between sessions, parents were expected to work on specific individualised programmes that were reviewed by the speech therapist at the end of each group. The group met weekly for an hour and 15 minutes. Each week the first five minutes was spent allowing the parents and carers to settle their children into the group room. The adults and children separated for about an hour. For about 10 minutes at the end of the session the parents joined the children's group for feedback time. The group relied on a number of items of equipment. These are listed in Box 15.3.

Box 15.3: Equipment for the feeding group

- Non-food (play) materials covering a range of tactile and olfactory experiences, for example wet and dry sand, Playdoh, cornflour mixed with water, bubbles, finger and face paints, aromatherapy oils, food colourings, chalks, paper of varying sizes and colours, fabric of varying textures
- Food (play) materials with a variety of textures, consistencies, colours, temperatures, flavours and smells
- Materials selected for whole group activities, such as icing biscuits, mixing deserts, making sandwiches
- A wide range of toys, ranging from baby toys to musical instruments
- Eating-associated equipment such as mouthable soft toys, a range of spoons, dishes, a toothbrush for each child, a range of cups
- TV and video equipment to record the children's progress and play back to the parents

---

The parents' group

The group aimed to approach parents' needs at a number of levels. These included the giving of instructions and advice, the encouragement of mutual support, and the facilitation of an understanding as to how their child's feeding difficulties may have developed and be maintained. In the first meeting the parents all introduced themselves and talked about their families, in particular about the child with the feeding difficulty (in practice this was not always confined to the disabled child). In the following weeks the group began with feedback from each family about the progress of their child. This would be followed by a discussion of any issues or theme that had arisen from the homework tasks or current issues within the family. This discussion, facilitated by the psychologist, would explore the factors that families considered helpful and those that hindered their progress with their child's feeding difficulties. Sometimes practical advice and problem-solving approaches were required, at other times the discussion would be more reflective and thoughtful. On occasion, the last half hour would be devoted to an invited professional. These 'speakers' would be invited at the request of the families, or would be selected for relevance to specific group difficulties.

Professional visiting speakers

Clinical nurse specialist

The clinical nurse specialist visited the group to talk about a range of aspects of feeding raised by the parents, including coughing and choking, focusing on both the causes of these conditions and their management. At other times, specialist nurses have talked about different types of gastrostomies and their management.

Occupational therapist and physiotherapist

The occupational therapist and physiotherapist talked about positioning and seating, specialist feeding equipment and gave practical advice on the process of feeding, tailored to each child. Where necessary, the relevant professional would visit the children's group to give advice to the professionals running this group.

Speech and language therapist

The speech and language therapist brought videofilm taken of the children within the feeding group to the parents' group to illustrate and focus on the nature and form of their children's interaction around the food-based activities. This information was then used as a basis for discussion and from this, a detailed observation of each child's verbal and non-verbal communicative behaviours was completed.

Portage/home visitors

The local portage team visited the parents' group to provide an 'experiential feeding experience'. They brought a range of food types, textures, flavours and temperatures, which the parents in pairs, one blindfolded, fed to each other on a range of feeding implements, e.g. metal and plastic spoons. The parents were able to experience feeding from the perspective of being unable to control the speed, quantity, variety or temperature of the food they received.

Dietician

The dietician visited the parents' group early on to ascertain the quantity of food the children were taking in and to develop an appropriate programme that both the professionals and parents could work with.

Paediatric dentist and dental hygienists

The dental team visited the parents' group to discuss a variety of dental issues, such as introducing the toothbrush, alternatives to the toothbrush, timing of feeding, order of presentation of foods and variety of foods.

Parent skills training

The clinical psychologist focused on parent skills training around eating, for example regularity of meal times and the eating environment. Parents were expected to keep records of their feeding behaviour, patterns and experiences as well as their children's. In practice, the educational aspect was not split from the supportive aspect of the group, rather, both aspects were drawn on in the course of each group meeting.

Support

The parents were encouraged, but not pressurised, to share their feelings, anxieties, concerns about any aspect of their management of the situation, their family relationships and their own feelings about feeding. Parents themselves offered ideas and support to each other. The psychologist worked at drawing out themes and helping parents think about how the feeding difficulties within the family developed and making links about how the difficulties were being maintained.

Issues and themes arising in the parents' group

The adults who attended the group were given between 30 minutes and an hour each week to think about issues to do with feeding. Over the course of facilitating the group in this form, a number of issues have consistently been raised within the adults' group.

Parents' own issues with eating

A frequent discussion within the group was related to the adults' own feelings and experiences with food. Often this would start with a discussion about the mess generated by attempts to feed their child. Mess was often described as unpleasant and unnecessary. Meal times were described as a necessity rather than an enjoyable family activity and got through as fast as possible, or with a distraction such as the television. Parents talked about understanding their child's fussiness as they themselves were fussy or picky about food. A regular discussion was that of how to generate a 'feeding-friendly' environment.

The child's special needs

Although not raised by the facilitator, in all the groups run to date, at some point parents themselves raised the issue of their child's disability. This took many forms, including discussions about what to say to strangers, how they were told the diagnosis, how they felt about their child growing up and comparisons with non-disabled siblings. Parents talked about the positives as well as the concerns with their child. On occasions some parents described how they felt ambivalent about the prospects of improvement in their child, that actually it was easier to continue feeding or tube-feeding their child rather than go through the experience of their child attempting to feed themselves. A frequently mentioned fear of change was of their child choking or gagging on food, and anxieties about parents physically harming their child by encouraging oral feeding.

Parents also focused on their child's physical disabilities and medical treatments. There was often an expression of feelings that to push their child after all they had been through was actually unfair or cruel. Through the process of thinking about these issues, parents were helped to become less anxious.

Family issues

Parents brought other issues to the group, the most common of which were family or marital issues. Often parents described feeling unsupported or blamed by the other parent/other family members for the child's difficulty. This tended to cause friction within the family or fed into the parents' already low self-esteem/mood. Over the course of the group, parents were encouraged to think about and track the issues within their families, and to monitor any effects on their child's feeding difficulty. Parents were good at helping each other notice or think about each other's family issues and at encouraging each other.

Frequent management issues

These included:

- advice around managing meal times. Often parents were separating their child's feeding from the rest of the family, feeding them in front of the TV, giving up easily when the child was refusing and providing an inconsistent feeding regime. Advice was given on providing a regular feeding pattern that approximated meal times and, where possible, when other family members were also eating
- advice around the communicative aspects of feeding. In several families the children had learnt to use vomiting, gagging, refusing or messing with food as a method of controlling their parents. The group often needed to focus on minimising the response to these behaviours and incorporating positive reinforcement for other areas of behaviour.

Children's group

The children's group aimed to provide a safe, child-centred environment, where the children were encouraged to develop normal eating experiences. Given that the majority of the children were deprived of normal eating experiences with roughly three quarters of the children being tube-fed, either via a nasogastric tube or gastrostomy, they required very basic food and non-food play.

In addition, because many of the children had chronic feeding difficulties, they had already progressed beyond the critical sensitive period, the optimum period for the introduction of semi-solid food. The aim was to enable the children to develop through the appropriate stages needed to attain oral feeding skills, such as desensitisation around the orofacial area, toleration of different textures, smells and other sensory stimuli on to toleration of different food consistencies and flavours. The desensitisation was extremely important for the children who had undergone numerous medical interventions, especially nasogastric tube insertion, as this leads to oral/orofacial hypersensitivity. Not surprisingly, this group of children often found any attempt at approaching their face or oral area aversive or unpleasant; that is, they had a learnt aversion to touch in these areas.

The group also focused on a systematic and controlled introduction of different food and non-food consistencies, temperatures, flavours and smells, thereby increasing the child's learning experiences. The slow, controlled introduction aimed to increase the child's tolerance in a positive and non-threatening way.

The group setting provided the impetus for the children to share experiences and to imitate each other's learning progress. Although they often played alone with a worker, they were often interested in what the others were doing. To facilitate this experience the group always included one whole group activity, such as making a pudding, decorating and icing biscuits, group hand and feet painting.

Each child had an individual programme, which included weekly progression of activities. As the group tended to be child led, these were encouraged, rather than dictated, and all the group facilitators were aware of each child's areas of need and targets.

The children's group format

The group started with the parents settling their children in (pre-school siblings were also allowed to attend) with a group 'sing-song'. The parents then left and the children were allowed to choose their own activities. The kinds of activities for the free play can be found in Box 15.4. Children were guided to engage in activities that showed a progression from week to week.

Box 15.4: Unstructured play activities for the children's group

- Foot, hand and, when the child was ready, face painting
- Dry and wet sand play
- Water play (sometimes bubbles and food dyes in the water)
- Music play
- Smelling activities, e.g. Playdoh with aromatherapy oils
- Collages with food, e.g. dry and cooked pasta, 100s and 1000s
- Thick liquid play, such as cornflour mixed with water
- Mouthable toys
- Construction toys

The play activities were organised so as to encourage the children's progress; for example face painting would be provided as an activity only after the children had mastered foot and hand painting. As part of the children's individual targets, and as whole/part group activities, a number of facilitator-led activities were introduced after the free play session. Some examples of these can be found in Box 15.5, selected to encourage development from week to week.

Box 15.5: Structured activities

- Hiding and seeking toys, hidden in food (e.g. flour, pasta, baked beans) and non-food (sand, water)
- Making sandwiches, puddings
- Blindfolding children (with their consent) and getting them to experience or guess different smells, then eventually flavours
- Guessing flavours of different liquids
- Tasting activities, such as presenting different flavours to children in a group
- Introduction to teethbrushing games

As with the free play, the structured play activities were introduced at the child's attainable level; that is, a child who had no oral feeding experience would not initially be introduced to thin liquids. Also the activities were structured around the child's cognitive abilities, so that more able and older children would have charts of achievement (e.g. obtaining pieces of a 'pie' to put together), whereas less cognitively able or younger children would have more immediate rewards, such as clapping, verbal praise, cuddles or other rewarding experiences.

Issues arising in the children's group

Separation anxiety

When the group was initially run, a structured 'settling in' period was not allowed for and many of the children found it very difficult to separate from their parents. This was not surprising, as often trips to the clinic have been aversive experiences for these children and they may especially fear being left. In addition, the parents were often anxious about leaving their children and expressed concern about the children not being able to look after themselves or manage being alone. Given the overall level of heightened anxiety at the beginning of the group, a formal 'settling in' period was introduced. This allowed the children to start activities in the presence of their parent, and for the parent to see what the child would be engaged in during the session. This had a positive effect on both parents' and children's ability to separate. In addition, because the two rooms were adjacent, it was possible for parents to hear if their child was unsettled or in distress. In such cases parents were encouraged to go and reassure their child before rejoining the parents' group.

Behavioural difficulties

A wide range of behavioural difficulties were observed, including vomiting, crying, gagging, retching and opting out. It was found that a firm, consistent approach to these behaviours, particularly ignoring the negative behaviours and rewarding positive behaviours, was the most helpful way of managing these difficulties.

Autistic children

During the time that the group ran a number of children attended who had been diagnosed as autistic. These children tended to have specific difficulties with feeding, particularly very restricted diets and extreme faddiness. They presented a specific challenge in the children's group, as on the whole they found being in a group difficult and the closed space restrictive. The most helpful way of managing their difficulties was to find an activity or object that they enjoyed and to ensure that it was always present for them.

Children's clothing

Interestingly, although the parents were made aware of the content of the children's group from the beginning of the group, they continued to bring their children wearing their 'best' clothes. This was managed by reinforcing the fact that the children would still be taking part in a wide range of 'messy' play experiences and the usual aprons were provided, with the parents often taking responsibility for cleaning their children at the end of the session.

Children with major physical disabilities

During the running of the group sessions a number of children with quite severe physical limitations attended. They needed considerable input from the occupational and physiotherapy services in terms of advice on positioning and the provision of appropriate equipment for feeding and play situations. They were also demanding of facilitator time, which led to the finding that, in order for the group to be successful, it was necessary to ensure a range of skills and ability levels in the children attending.

Older children

There was quite a range of children attending the various groups that were run, i.e. occasionally a mix of both pre-school and school-aged children. This difficulty was managed through the provision of specific and individually tailored programmes that used the same activities presented in a manner more fitting for their cognitive abilities, e.g. achievement charts, scavenger hunts and guessing games. This meant that each group session had to be carefully planned to meet the needs of a wide range of abilities.

Outcome measures

A number of measures were set up from the beginning of the group. These included: feedback from parents, both informally and formally through a questionnaire; feedback from the therapists working with the children as to their progress; and finally, where possible, from other professionals working with the families.

The benefits described by parents included:

- a reduction in the use of tubes for feeding
- a reduction in the anxiety around feeding
- a greater understanding of the feeding process
- a greater understanding of the emotional and behavioural aspects of feeding
- recognised improvements in the children, e.g. quantity and variety of foodstuffs accepted orally increased
- reduced unwanted behaviour (e.g. throwing) at meal times
- appreciation of sharing concerns with other parents.

Areas where parents expressed dissatisfaction included:

- the number of group sessions (parents wanted more)
- the disruption to the day
- not enough time during the group
- a wish for more home-based treatment.

From the facilitators' perspective, there were considerable improvements in the children:

- increased tolerance of tactile experiences (both food and non-food)
- acceptance of a wider range of food consistencies
- decrease in level of anxiety at 'meal times'
- interest in food as a non-threatening play experience
- more successful communicative interactions between parents and their children.

A case example of child and parent: Andrea and Mrs K

Andrea

Andrea was referred to the feeding group by her portage worker and her specialist community nurse. Andrea was a two and a half year old girl who had been diagnosed at birth as having Down's syndrome. Andrea was born with severe medical difficulties, both gastrooesophageal and cardiac. She had been placed in special care from birth, and she received neonatal surgery and remained in special care until aged eight months, when she was returned home. Owing to her oesophageal stricture, she required nasogastric feeding. In addition, when oral feeding was introduced it was discovered that she aspirated thin liquids, so oral feeding was discontinued at this time. She had received numerous medical interventions during the last two and a half years. At the time of the referral Andrea already had a gastrostomy tube *in situ*. Her paediatrician was now recommending a move to oral feeding. Her mother, Mrs K, had tried to introduce smooth semi-solids. However, Andrea had a tendency to vomit or gag with these.

Mrs K

Mrs K was a single parent, and had two older children, both boys (aged seven and nine). Her marriage had broken down around the time of Andrea's birth and the portage worker was concerned that Mrs K had not got over the break-up of the marriage and was associating this with Andrea's diagnosis. Mrs K was keen to attend a parents' group as she talked of being isolated with her difficulties and that too much was expected of her with Andrea's feeding difficulties.

At the initial meeting, Mrs K described having difficulties managing Andrea's behaviour, particularly Andrea's gagging behaviour, which she felt was an indication that Andrea was not entirely ready for oral feeding. We also learnt that Andrea's brothers complained about the mess that Andrea made when she tried to feed her and that it just seemed too much effort when her nutritional needs could be met by her gastrostomy tube-feeds.

Andrea's feeding group experience

Initially Andrea found it difficult to separate from her mother and she cried for long periods. However, if the crying was ignored and she was presented with distracting activities, she quickly stopped. Initially Andrea was presented with non-food activities to enable her to feel safe. These included tactile experiences, such as playing with toys in water and finding toys buried in sand. Andrea enjoyed these activities and especially liked getting the attention and positive reinforcement that was associated. After three groups it was possible to introduce food play. She did not like touching food materials such as cooked spaghetti and baked beans (anything that was not smooth); however, when it was combined with a task that she could achieve such as finding a small toy, she would attempt it.

Andrea was then ready to move on to tasting experiences. She was offered different tastes on a plastic animal toy. Initially she tried to get the worker to try the tastes. She was very engaging with this and was able to distract a worker's attention. However, when the worker persisted, Andrea would indicate no, by shaking her head. She would not actually move away from the food and with gentle persuasion she would eventually attempt tastes. Over the course of the next few weeks, a record was gathered of the different kinds of tastes that Andrea liked and did not like. She had clear preferences for savoury tastes (Marmite, tomato ketchup, salty flavours, smooth peanut butter, tuna paste) and was not keen on sweet flavours (chocolate, honey, yoghurt, fruit purée). After 16 group sessions she was accepting small amounts of a range of puréed foods and was demonstrating a real interest in thickened liquids.

Mrs K's group experience

When Mrs K joined the group she was very positive about the prospect of change. She talked openly about feeling isolated and was visibly pleased that others shared this. Her optimism diminished in the third week, when she came in complaining that Andrea was not eating and that there was no point in coming as things wouldn't change. In discussion with the group she was able to talk about how difficult she found the homework tasks as she felt that things were moving too quickly for Andrea, who she described as her 'little baby' who had been through so much already. She then talked about her anger at professionals in their handling of Andrea's diagnosis and early care. She and her husband had been told separately and they had not been able to see Andrea until a day after her birth. Initially she blamed the hospital for the breakdown in her marital relationship, saying that 'things might have worked out if I hadn't spent so much time with Andrea in hospital'. Later on during the group she acknowledged that the relationship was breaking down prior to the birth of Andrea. This acknowledgement allowed Mrs K to shift her perception of Andrea from blaming her (and then needing to see her as precious to alleviate the bad feelings/guilt this caused) to seeing Andrea's role in the marital split more realistically.

In the sixth week, the speech and language therapist visited the group with video clips from the children's group showing Andrea sampling different flavours. Mrs K expressed surprise, saying that she couldn't believe that Andrea would be able to do this. She became despondent about this, saying that others were having more success than she. The group were able to help Mrs K see Andrea's developments as positive, they were able to consider that the developments were in part *because* the workers were not so 'emotionally involved'.

Andrea's change in behaviour was then enough to encourage Mrs K to renew her efforts on the homework tasks. By the eighth week Mrs K talked with pride about how Andrea had eaten two spoonfuls of puréed food without gagging or vomiting.

Conclusion

The feeding group programme combined treatments at a number of levels (physical, social and psychological). Although only a small number have been through this programme since its inception (22 children), of these 16 demonstrated improvements in the amount of food taken orally, representing a 72% success rate. Five others showed some improvements in their ability to tolerate facial touch, even though their oral consumption did not change. One child's oral consumption decreased. This appeared to be associated with increased family difficulties. In addition the project received a quality of service award from the local healthcare trust, as it was judged to be 'innovative' and helpful.

References

Alexander R (1987) Oral-motor treatment for infants and young children with cerebral palsy. *Seminars in Speech and Language.* **8**: 87–100.

Chamberlin JL, Henry MM, Roberts JD, Sapsford AL and Courtney SE (1991) An infant and toddler feeding group program. *American Journal of Occupational Therapy.* **45**(10): 907–11.

Dale N (1996) *Working with Families of Children with Special Needs: partnership and practice.* Routledge, London.

Daws D (1993) Feeding problems and relationship difficulties: therapeutic work with parents and infants. *Journal of Child Psychotherapy.* **19**(2): 69–83.

Gisel EG (1990) The role of the occupational therapist in the evaluation and care of infants and children with feeding problems. *Journal of Neurologic Rehabilitation.* **4**(2): 111–14.

Griggs CA, Jones PM and Lee RE (1989) Videofluoroscopic investigations of feeding disorders of children with multiple handicap. *Developmental Medicine and Child Neurology.* **31**(3): 303–8.

Luiselli JK (1994) Oral feeding treatment of children with chronic food refusal and multiple developmental disabilities. *American Journal on Mental Retardation.* **98**(5): 646–55.

Luiselli JK and Luiselli TE (1995) A behaviour analysis approach toward chronic food refusal in children with gastrostomy-tube dependency. *Topics in Early Childhood Special Education.* **15**(1): 1–18.

Menzies-Lyth I (1988) *Containing Anxieties in Institutions. Selected Essays*, vol 1. Free Association Books, London.

Neill S and Irvine B (1994) Multidisciplinary Team Feeding Difficulties Audit. Redbridge Health Care Trust.

Reilly S and Skuse D (1992) Characteristics and management of feeding problems of young children with cerebral palsy. *Developmental Medicine and Child Neurology.* **34**(5): 379–88.

Rosenthal SR, Sheppard JJ and Lotze M (1995) *Dysphagia and the Child with Developmental Disabilities.* Singular Publishing, California.

Wolf LS and Glass RP (1992) *Feeding and Swallowing Disorders in Infancy. Assessment and Management.* Therapy Skill Builders, Tucson, Arizona.

CHAPTER 16

A community feeding service

Jacqui Mitchell and Katie Thomas

Introduction

This chapter covers the background and practical issues involved in setting up a community feeding service. It discusses the context and the rationale behind the service together with the evolving multidisciplinary involvement, outlining how objectives were established and how the service was 'formalised' through business planning and dedicated funding. Future directions and developments are also discussed in the light of experiences and progress to date.

The community feeding service is a developing provision and needs continued energy and time to keep the momentum going. The service spans two hospital trusts and includes both inpatient and community services. The professionals involved in the feeding service are drawn from the health service, as well as social services, education and general practice.

The aim of the community service is to provide as cohesive and consistent a service as possible to all children and their families. It is facilitated by having a central referral point, a comprehensive card index of all relevant children and a forum to generate discussion on managing the children's needs among the many professionals who work with them.

Establishing the need for a service

Many different professionals are involved with children with problematic feeding behaviour. As is probably the case in most areas, idiosyncrasies in provision, policy and service structure do not make for consistencies in approaching feeding problems. This situation is not helped by the fragmentation of healthcare services. In many hospital services, those professionals involved in the early stages of the feeding service described find themselves straddling more than one service-providing trust or hospital. Not only does this impair communication and collaborative working but it also means that in some cases there are organisational impediments to working together. When special schools staff, social workers, GPs and health visitors are included, the picture becomes even more complicated. Treatment of feeding difficulties seems to be dependent on whoever happens to identify problems.

The idea of promoting a multidisciplinary approach to this area of work developed slowly and was a culmination of several different strands of work, the impetus being a set of circumstances rather than a plan. One of the initiating factors was a seminar given by Hodges and Harris (*see* Chapter 15). Following this, a number of professionals were approached to discuss the possibility of setting up a specialist feeding team. Visits were then made to other centres to gain more insight into the services they offered. This gave the opportunity of consolidating ideas and theories while also facilitating teamwork. Through talking to colleagues it became apparent that children with similar problems were being referred to dietetics, speech therapy and the child mental health services. Sometimes referrals were made to all three services, suggesting that more consistency and coordination were vital. Although referrals were made on a seemingly ad hoc basis, the general feeling was that each service had specialist and complementary knowledge to contribute to the assessment and treatment process.

Audit of cases

The initial step was to determine the extent of multiprofessional involvement and types of feeding problems via an audit of current cases. Those included were children who presented with feeding difficulties due to:

- health-related feeding problems
- tube-feeding
- problems with feeding management
- behavioural problems or social difficulties giving rise to feeding problems.

Departments and personnel contacted included the community paediatrician, community paediatric nurses, speech and language therapists, child psychiatry, clinical psychology, dietetics, school nurses in special schools, physiotherapists, pre-school service for special needs and health visitors. Seventy-three children were identified initially, some in contact with up to five professionals at the same time. Leading on from this, a talk was given to health visitors to discuss the aims of a feeding service and the children who may benefit from it. The data collected from both the case audit and from the response from professionals demonstrated a need for the service.

A combination of data gathering, visiting, discussion and liaison with other professionals, and information on the causes of feeding problems (Chatoor *et al.* 1984) suggested that the service should have the following issues at its core:

- practical sessions with desensitisation and suitable stimulation
- support for parents
- prevention of chronic feeding problems for those starting on nasogastric/ gastrostomy feeding at a young age
- support for a planned, programmed return to oral feeding.

Promoting multidisciplinary involvement

A multidisciplinary seminar was planned to present issues and promote further discussion, this time around the practicalities of setting up such a service. The subsequent day-long seminar was divided into a morning of papers and an afternoon of workshops with discussions around recommendations for further work. The general consensus of opinion was that a cohesive approach was lacking and it was decided that a steering group should be set up, with one of its aims being the generation of a business plan to formalise the service. A core group of professionals was therefore established to liaise regularly about general methods and training strategies, as well as about specific children referred to the service. The seminar provided considerable impetus to the service initiative.

Discovering a dilemma: does having the technology mean that it gets used more?

Our own research showed that the provision of home tube-feeding continued to escalate and that this was perhaps made easier by the availability of an excellent community paediatric nursing service. The dilemma existed in the use of technological methods to the exclusion of other natural methods. Tube-feeding can be started relatively easily, and pressure is taken off parents and professionals when children tolerate it and gain weight. This brings with it the responsibility for giving parents and children the support to encourage oral feeding. The results of our survey suggested strongly that a network needed to be in place to prevent over-treatment through enteral nutrition at the expense of oral nutrition. It seems important to balance the available expertise and technology with support, encouragement and suitable advice designed to shorten the length of time a child needs to be tube-fed. Much time and effort should be put into the encouragement of parents to feed their children orally and not to rely on tube-feeding instead of eating (Chatoor *et al.* 1997).

Overall objectives of an integrated service

With the material from other centres, feedback from the audit, the data about specific children seen locally obtained by the questionnaire and the research into numbers, the following objectives were formulated.

Early intervention

Early intervention was seen as being of great importance, especially considering that problems of poor feeding behaviour may become entrenched and very difficult to help. This is especially relevant with children born prematurely, where feeding and weight gain are of such great importance while the baby is in hospital and where parents may feel vulnerable when the child is first discharged home (Gardner and Hagedorn 1991a,b). First-line helpers, GPs and health visitors, are of prime importance in this role, and hopefully training for these professionals is to be part of the overall service, as well as input into special care baby units in hospital. It is hoped to provide a 'fast response' service to parents when their children are first identified as having difficulties.

Preventative work

A need was identified to develop preventative work with parents, to provide information about good feeding behaviour at an early stage in their child's life (Duniz *et al.* 1996) and to have consultation with health visitors in relation to advice they give. Most children develop faddy eating at some point and there exists a clear need to identify when the child is having above-average difficulties in feeding.

Comprehensive range of interventions

Comprehensive therapy for these families is necessary so that both parents and professionals know where to go for help when they have exhausted their resources. A point of contact for children and their parents needs to be provided that enables them to access a range of expertise in how to manage children with very problematic feeding behaviour (Daws 1994). Advice the feeding team may give to parents is not always 'common sense' advice. For example, recommendations that children be allowed initially to eat what they like without regard for nutritional balance is contrary to parental expectation. Similarly, reassuring parents that 'no food is bad food', suggesting that children feed regularly through the day and advising parents never to force or cajole the child often seems paradoxical. They are difficult strategies for parents and carers to implement so they need support and encouragement. There is a need for parents to share some of their frustrations and a group setting, where they could discuss different management ideas with professionals and other parents, was felt to be beneficial. Rosenthal *et al.* (1995) describe how social support is crucial. Similarly, groups for children were also felt to be useful. This is covered in more detail in Chapter 15. Chamberlin *et al.* (1991) have described a similar support group.

Increasing professional knowledge and skills

Another objective of an integrated service is to increase the knowledge and skills of the staff, and to increase cooperation and collaboration among professionals. Early on in the process, research revealed that few other agencies offered an integrated service along the lines of our blueprint, so any help from others was gratefully received. It was clear to all those working in this field that different professionals had different baselines when dealing with children who would not eat. The understanding of each other's perspective is crucial when attempting to help. Medical intervention is very different to psychological intervention, and in some cases the two seem to conflict. The encouragement of openness and debate within the core group, and in case conference discussions, is essential to prevent workers pulling against each other. In some cases the only solution is to agree to disagree and attempt a working plan for the immediate future. The overall aim is to help the child to achieve a normal eating pattern and to work towards this in a constructive manner.

Training

Training is seen to be very high priority. There is a need for those in the field to be trained, while also providing continued education for other professionals. Valuable experience can be gained by visiting other units, particularly those which have developed integrated services. It has been possible to use professionals from within the trust to provide training locally. The resources of other professions have been of immense help in this respect, and the team continues to refine its approaches through their expertise.

Summary of service

One of the recommendations from the audit day was to write a business plan for presentation to management, so that a children's feeding team could be developed. Convincing professionals dealing with patient care that a service was needed was not difficult. However, convincing budget holders to part with money and persuading them that it is money well spent was quite a different matter. To provide the kind of service described, additional resources are necessary. Reorganisation of work offered the possibility of starting a weekly feeding clinic, but additional resources were required to provide a good service with sufficient professional and administrative back-up.

In writing a business plan it is necessary to justify to the management that the recommended proposal is worthwhile and cost-effective. Every locality has its own specific needs; what follows is the business plan in a specific area.

Strategic planning and establishing organisational frameworks

First the plan was to have one point of referral with a core group of professionals who would look at the referral and coordinate the service to the child. This led to the second proposal, which was a feeding clinic that the core team would facilitate. This would be run on a weekly basis to develop a planned, staged return to normal, oral feeding in children whose food refusal had become chronic. Support and teaching for the parents would be an integral part of the feeding clinic. There would also be education and information for other professionals and a feeding forum for those dealing with children with feeding difficulties.

Finding measurable targets for gauging progress is difficult but important. The following were considered possible:

- conducting user surveys of the service
- looking at referral rates and numbers of children who are resistant to change, which should fall if education and giving advice are effective
- purchasers' feedback regarding coherency and effectiveness of the service
- reductions in the length of time children are on tube-feeding at home.

To achieve these goals there are human resource implications. For instance, we found that setting up a weekly feeding clinic of one full afternoon per week required two nursery nurses, with one extra team member to run the group. One trained professional is needed to lead a discussion group for parents, relating to their children's difficulties, and staff are needed to run a drop-in service for both parents and professionals, who can telephone or drop in for advice on any kind of feeding problem with children. Alongside this there is the time of the professionals in the core group meeting for at least one and a half hours per month or more as the need arises. Fast response and a home assessment service for those children where there is a possibility that tube-feeding may be needed require additional time commitments. Finally, secretarial support is necessary to make appointments, organise meetings, type minutes, collate resource material and undertake other support functions such as preparing acetates for presentations and to deal with the distribution of resources.

Savings can be made in several ways:

- streamlining the service to prevent duplication by different professionals
- highlighting the need for training at the primary healthcare level to give early, skilled intervention to prevent some of the severe feeding problems
- reducing the cost of tube-feeding.

If both the length of time that a child is tube-fed and the number of children starting on tube-feeding are reduced, then some considerable saving could be made.

Having looked at the cost implications, the business plan then went on to identify what issues were hindering the progress of treating children with feeding difficulties, and what improvements could be made.

In line with the objectives previously discussed, a feeding service would address the following important issues:

- a single central referral point for feeding problems
- early intervention
- management of complex feeding problems
- coordination and supervision of personnel in less severe cases
- training of other professionals
- production of literature for professionals and parents
- setting up of a feeding clinic for chronic cases
- consistent advice on feeding issues.

The business plan also covered other topics, including the principal services that were currently involved with the children who had feeding difficulties. It described each professional's involvement and how their contribution to the therapy helps support the child and the family. Assessing current performance against targets was not possible, as no targets had been set on these issues internally. However, from informal discussions with health professionals and the interest and enthusiasm expressed at the multidisciplinary seminar, it was apparent that there was an urgent demand for a coherent service together with in-service training.

It has to be assumed that once the service is promoted and becomes more widely known, the number of referrals will increase. Therefore, to continue to develop the service further resources will be required. A three- to five-year forecast is not easy to make. It is hoped that by this time all children who have a feeding difficulty, whether the root cause is physical or psychological, will be able to receive some form of assessment and help in relation to their feeding.

Client satisfaction

Satisfaction for the patients is an important criterion, which should be highlighted. If the feeding service achieves its objective, children should get a quicker, more effective service. The child's problems should be dealt with earlier, as front-line professionals will have information and training, which should go some way towards preventing difficulties becoming intractable. Also patients should be allocated more quickly to the most appropriate worker, thus reducing waiting time.

Accommodation

The final consideration on the business plan was the need for accommodation.

The team needs to have a central referral point, with secretarial support, appropriate office furniture and a computer. Computer software would be needed for collating information for purchasers and clinical information for research and audit purposes, as well as for the production of literature for internal information and training. A small group of rooms where meetings can be held and files and other resource materials kept would be ideal.

The feeding group itself needs the use of a playroom with a variety of play and food equipment. Play materials need to be appropriate, with emphasis on tactile play, facilities for water and sand play, and somewhere to prepare food. This needs to be permanent as it is very difficult moving play materials. Often one planned activity will move naturally on to another unplanned one, so the room needs permanence to allow for this spontaneity. It is also necessary to have a meeting room for parents, with facilities for tea and coffee making.

Core group

The aim of implementing the core group is to improve communication between professionals and enable all those involved to work together as a coordinated team. Working together as a multidisciplinary team is essential for quality of patient care, successful management of the problem and the cost-effectiveness of the service.

The core team includes representatives from clinical psychology services, dietetics, community paediatric nursing, speech and language therapy, and medicine (e.g. community paediatrician). It was felt that a medical screening of all children should first be provided, with one or more of the core team then seeing children for assessment and therapy, as appropriate.

The core group meets monthly and has two functions. First, it discusses referrals to the team and ensures communication is maintained. Second, it acts as a forum where all professionals involved in the field can come for formal presentations and discussion.

The core group aims to write literature and provide education and training for professionals involved. All members of the core team will have a special interest in feeding difficulties in children. They will, however, need to maintain a level of expertise by in-service training and by attending appropriate courses.

Moving the service forward

With the setting up of an integrated service, further developments are anticipated. There is a need to educate parents, to prevent feeding difficulties arising and for all professions to give consistent informed advice. The pre-school service, teachers, helpers and school nurses in special schools all give support, therapy, help with feeding technique and psychological input, as do ward staff and the special care baby unit. The need for discussions with each other on these issues is important. Further, it is becoming increasingly apparent that feeding difficulties are often associated with premature births. Working with special care baby units in this area should be a further step in preventing feeding difficulties (Gardner and Hagedorn 1991a,b).

Where children are of school age or attend a special school, and where visiting a weekly feeding clinic is not appropriate, the team has run a feeding clinic in the school. The benefit is to increase communication with the school. The downside is that parents are less likely to attend the clinic. Taking the clinic to the school may be practically more difficult but building confidence, cooperation and a consistent way of working by professionals must be seen as of immense value.

Taking a clinic to a health centre is a further possibility and provides easier access for the parents. When dealing with any new approaches, adequate briefing is essential. All staff need to understand the principles behind the clinic and there should be debriefing at the end so that ideas and observations can be shared and discussed.

The overall purpose of these developments is to reach as many children as possible and as early as possible before feeding problems have become entrenched, and to ensure that professionals are giving consistent advice leading to a well-coordinated approach.

Summary

It can be seen from this chapter that the fundamental principle behind setting up a multidisciplinary community feeding team is to provide fora for discussion and opportunities to share ideas, methods of treatment and work practices. We established that it was essential that the service find time to keep communications open between all professionals and to work together so that methods of practice are consistent.

It has been shown how the multidisciplinary seminar was instrumental in providing opportunities for sharing experiences, information and ideas and how the core team then continued this momentum. The feeding clinic provided the practical therapy for these children and the business plan was the means of developing it so that our objectives could be met.

Looking back, it can be seen that the service developed as a result of a series of events and interested personnel, together with the growing awareness by various professionals of the increasing number of children with chronic feeding difficulties. The development of the service in another area will be defined by existing resources and personnel and will not necessarily consist of the same format as described above. However, it is hoped that the ideas and developments that have been experienced will go some way towards stimulating the setting up of similar services elsewhere.

Appendix: Case histories of children attending the feeding clinic

Murkah

Age when referred to child and family mental health: three years.

Murkah was born at 28 weeks gestation. His mother needed to feed him every 1.5 hours, and he took 45 minutes to feed. In discussions it became apparent that his mother was depressed, but this had not been recognised or treated, and special care nurses came out daily to weigh Murkah. His mother remembered this time as one of constant feeding, and feared he would die if he did not eat/feed well.

Murkah would eat nothing voluntarily, but was force-fed Weetabix and rusk. Murkah often vomited all his food.

His mother's depression continued; she was not supported by her husband, who had great difficulty coming to terms with his 'less than perfect' baby, and who opted out rather than face the issues.

Murkah was a child with severe learning difficulties, and has only recently received help from education and other support services. His mother felt uncomfortable both asking for and accepting help, and as Murkah was her first child she was unsure of 'what is normal'. This led to delays in the family receiving help and they had no counselling in relation to Murkah's handicap.

As with nearly all children with chronic non-feeding behaviour, the event that precipitated the problem is not necessarily what maintains it, and there were a number of issues relevant to the continuance of the problem.

With Murkah the following factors were significant:

- his mother was depressed and had been since Murkah's birth
- both parents, but especially his father, found it hard to accept that Murkah had permanent learning difficulties and would need special education
- the marriage was under strain since his father had given up work to attend full-time university and his mother had to give up work to care for Murkah.

The feeding group offered a two-pronged approach, providing play for Murkah, and advice and support for his mother. The group, run by two nursery nurses, concentrated on giving tactile experiences with a variety of textures and materials. There was 'food time', where children were encouraged to experiment with food and get involved with spreading and mixing. Eating was an added bonus, never forced or coerced. Murkah's mother was encouraged to adopt this easy manner, to be more relaxed around food, to overcome her need to wipe him clean and to enjoy the experience.

She was given an opportunity to talk without Murkah, to observe him through the screen and to share some of her frustrations. Nutritional supplements were prescribed, which she could give if he did not eat. This reduced her anxiety and hence her need to force-feed.

Murkah was initially very tactile defensive, would not touch food, would guide his mother's hand to the crisps for her to feed him and would wipe his hands if they became wet, salty or sticky. Progress was very slow, his learning difficulty meant his concentration was poor and he needed close supervision with all activity.

In parallel with this, the family was beginning to receive appropriate educational help. Murkah was given some respite care and a baby-sitting scheme was implemented. In addition, staff from the nursery did some intensive behaviour management with his mother at home to help her manage his behaviour, especially his sleep.

At the time of writing, Murkah is in school full-time, is eating voluntarily and managing a full meal most of the time. He is no longer on food supplements and force-feeding is a thing of the past.

Gill

Age when referred: two years three months.

Gill was the youngest of three children; her mother was a lone parent, separated following a violent relationship with the children's father.

Gill was a small child and had very bad asthma, needing hospital admission several times. She was seen regularly by the paediatrician to follow up her healthcare and he often expressed concern about her weight. She grew slowly and was quite small, but there had been no concerns about her development or her eating. Her mother reported she had had a good appetite; indeed she used to eat cottage pie and roast potatoes with the family.

Gill was admitted to hospital following an infection, pneumonia and asthma, and spent the Christmas period in hospital. Her eating on the ward was poor, so as soon as she was well enough for discharge a nasogastric tube was put in so she could be discharged home. Her mother was in agreement with this; she was anxious for Gill to be home with her brothers. She was referred to the feeding team four months later for a behavioural feeding problem.

Gill was still being followed up for her chest problems and at these appointments she was always weighed. Her mother reported how she would feel sick while waiting, in case Gill had not gained weight. Her mother found the tube reassuring, as the pressure was taken away from her at meal times, but she was worried that Gill was not eating.

There were again a number of issues affecting non-feeding behaviour:

- overnight feeding meant her tummy was full and her need for food during the day was lessened
- the tube in her nose increased the sensitivity around her mouth and throat
- her mother was anxious, alone and unsupported at home; her worries about weight gain led her to create tensions and scenes at meal times, which were not conducive to her child eating well
- her mother found mess difficult and was in the habit of wiping her daughter during feeding so she did not make a mess, thus removing some of the control from Gill.

The feeding group offered play and social activity for Gill, with emphasis on her being in control and getting messy. For her mother it was an opportunity to share feelings and frustrations, to look at different ways of managing Gill and to help her reduce some of her own behaviours that were militating against Gill's return to oral feeding.

At the time of writing Gill has been off tube-feeding for 18 months and is eating well. She is still very small and does not gain weight easily, but remains in good health.

Doug

Age when referred: three years.

Doug was born at 25 weeks gestation and had both breathing and feeding difficulties in hospital. He had lung damage and suffered with asthma, having only half of one lung functioning. He was discharged home aged four months, but needed considerable hospital back-up because of his physical health problems. His mother was a lone parent, coming late to parenthood at 40.

There were several occasions where Doug had life-threatening illnesses, and more than once his mother described the fear he may have died. As a small baby he took a very long time to feed and a pattern of forcing him developed. He would vomit on any lump, however soft, and would gag frequently. His mother would then offer something else, often needing to liquidise it before offering it to him. By the time he was referred to the team, he was eating nothing voluntarily and drinking only small amounts.

Doug was a very small child, thin and wasted-looking, with odd developmental traits and many obsessions. He was diagnosed with Asperger's syndrome at five years.

There were several initiating factors to Doug's feeding problem, not least his very poor physical health and his slow and uneven development. The following were relevant factors that maintained his erratic feeding:

- Doug's mother agreed that her world revolved around him and she found it very difficult to ignore his non-eating
- his physical health was poor, he had bad asthma and regularly needed antibiotics. This affected his appetite
- with Doug's diagnosis of Asperger's syndrome, his obsessive behaviour fell into place. He found change very distressing, panicked if routines were altered and so would not accept the introduction of new food or something unfamiliar.

The feeding group offered Doug an opportunity to mix with other children and to manage change in a very calm and easy setting. For Doug's mother, there was social contact with other parents, some of whose children were 'worse' than hers, and an opportunity to discuss management.

Progress with these children is very slow and small changes need high-lighting, otherwise parents quickly become disheartened and return to old habits, feeling that nothing is being gained. Parents need constant reminders of how things were and how far they have come. Sharing experiences with other parents who are a little further ahead has, in our experience, proved to be most valuable.

Doug was prescribed supplements for the daytime, so his mother did not need to force-feed him. As the force-feeding stopped, his vomiting stopped, with the result that emotionally everyone felt better.

At the time of writing, Doug is in full-time school. The staff are learning to manage his odd behaviour and have had considerable advice and support with his feeding. Doug was found to be extremely gifted with words and numbers, and good at obeying written instructions. Writing down what was expected of him proved helpful in getting him to eat. This is an interesting example of using a child's skills and allowing them to remain in control. He is now beginning to try new foods and eat reasonable amounts voluntarily.

Angelique

Age when referred: one year six months.

Angelique was diagnosed as suffering from fetal alcohol syndrome. She had been small since birth, with height and weight below the third centile. With the continual concern about her failing to thrive, she was given a nasogastric tube when she was 13 months old. Her parents were devoted to her; she was the youngest of eight children living at home, but with a chaotic family life, it was difficult to get an accurate history of feeding and eating behaviour.

On assessment, Angelique was gaining most nutrition from the tube; she was fed overnight and initially the pump was turned off for an hour at 3 am to prevent vomiting. She drank from both cup and bottle, but usually had milk in the day from a bottle; if this was not finished it was given via the tube. She did put food to her mouth and was less reticent than other children to try tastes; she showed no sign of aversion. However, her oral intake was very small, especially of fluids.

There were a number of factors present within the family that were affecting her poor feeding pattern:

- Angelique was the youngest child at home, who was regarded by the rest of the family as a precious child, and most of the time she was allowed to do as she pleased. Her parents acknowledged that she 'ruled them all'
- her parents were both alcoholics, routines at home were haphazard, and many older children and relatives were responsible for caring for Angelique
- she had a small appetite and was full after being fed overnight. She had little time for food during the day. Her parents felt safe knowing they could give her food by tube, because they enjoyed the security it gave
- the family was very clean, almost to the point of obsession; the house was spotless in spite of the children, and Angelique would not tolerate mess or stickiness. She would not drink from her bottle if anyone else had touched it, and would insist it was cleaned.

In the feeding group we concentrated on the social skills and on encouraging Angelique to get messy while playing. She made considerable progress with this and gained from the social contact with other children as she did not go to nursery. We also helped her mother to be relaxed about food and food play, letting Angelique choose what to eat and what to play with. The clinic time was also used to assess how much Angelique was eating, to look at her overnight feeds and to make any relevant changes. We encouraged her parents to leave the tube out during the daytime so Angelique did not have the sensitisation around her face and throat.

Progress with Angelique went well. Her oral intake increased, she started taking a lot more fluids, she came off the tube and she was less tactile defensive. She was taking supplements to increase her nutritional intake. At the time of writing, it was hoped that she would attend pre-school nursery.

Krish

Age when referred: five years.

Krish had been known to paediatrics and dietetics almost since birth. He had severe learning and physical difficulties, and attended special school since he was four years old.

He was born addicted to butane gas lighter fuel, used by his mother throughout the pregnancy. When he was a week old, his mother left. He was cared for by his father, and there were concerns about his growth and development since he was a tiny baby.

He was diagnosed as non-organic failure to thrive in his first year. At 13 months Krish was given a nasogastric tube, which he did not tolerate well. He hated it being passed and was often sick.

Following many case conferences and discussions, he was given a gastrostomy in summer 1997 aged almost five years. He had minimal oral intake, would drink milk and juice, but did not appear to chew. He would eat yoghurt if chased with a spoon. There was no evidence that he had been force-fed.

His initial feeding problem was probably a result of some brain damage prior to birth, a possible injury when he was six weeks old and a parent who had struggled to care for his child. There were a number of factors that affected his continued non-eating:

- he was highly sensitised by the experience of nasogastric feeding, he used to vomit and, because of the distress, it was thought his father did not always put the tube in
- his father was quite disorganised at home, did not have a cooker and did not always offer Krish food at meal times
- his father was always anxious about asking for help. He was brought up in care, felt he was failed by professionals and was mistrustful of motives when health and social services got involved.

The biggest problem when working with Krish was trying to include his father in the work. The group was taken to Krish's special school, where there were three children with similar difficulties. Six sessions were run, involving school staff in the work. Krish was very tactile defensive, he would gag at the *sight* of wet pasta and was reluctant to touch anything sticky or wet. He would not put any food in his mouth, so work involved play with toothbrushes and lollies, and other activities designed to help him overcome some of his fear. His learning difficulty made progress slow and without his father being part of the process it was difficult for Krish to move on.

At the time of writing, Krish is eating yoghurt on his own and his father is cooperating with the oral feeding programme. A programme between school, home and the paediatric nursing service has been agreed, with everyone using the same methods. An important aspect of this has been bolus feeding in the day, to simulate meal times. The programme was reviewed regularly and his father was able to see the advantages of helping Krish towards more normal feeding behaviour.

Mosha

Age when referred: two years four months.

Mosha had been known to the pre-school health services since his discharge from hospital aged 16 months. He was extremely ill for a long time in his first year, and more than once his parents were prepared for his death. He was a very precious child at home, usually getting his own way and was very pampered. He was the youngest of seven children.

He was born with a diaphragmatic hernia and was fed entirely by nasogastric tube until just prior to his discharge from hospital, aged 16 months. He ate almost nothing orally, although he would take a cup and put food in his mouth. He had no ability to move the food from the front to the back of his mouth, so any food put in would be spat out. He was given a gastrostomy and was thriving; his weight gain was good and his health seemed stable.

There were a number of precipitating factors to Mosha's feeding difficulties: his very poor health, his inability to feed orally, his slow weight gain and his parents' anxieties about his general health and well being. The following were issues:

- Mosha was fed via a gastrostomy tube overnight, his nutritional needs were met and he was not hungry
- developmentally he had an immature chew and swallow, and so he was not able to eat normally
- he was the centre of attention at home and the family did nothing to upset him, so there were not many controls and boundaries
- the family was so pleased he was well and thriving that they did not have a strong need to change the pattern by introducing food, which they felt would upset him.

Work with Mosha was hindered by the family's ambivalence and the fact that his mother did not speak English. It was planned to have a translator in the group, but the family did not attend regularly. The speech therapy assessment indicated that Mosha needed some basic help with moving food around his mouth and the team did not have regular access to such speech and language therapy help.

At the time of writing, Mosha is still fed via his tube and no progress had been made with his oral feeding.

References

Chamberlin JL, Henry MM, Roberts JD, Sapsford AL and Courtney SE (1991) An infant and toddler feeding group program. *American Journal of Occupational Therapy.* **45**(10): 907–11.

Chatoor I, Schaefer S, Dickson L and Egan J (1984) A developmental approach to feeding disturbances: failure to thrive and growth disorders in young children. *Pediatric Annals.* **13**(11).

Chatoor I, Hirsh K and Persinger M (1997) Facilitating internal regulation of eating: a treatment model for infantile anorexia. *Infants and Young Children.* **9**(4): 12–22.

Daws D (1994) Family relationships and infant feeding problems. *Health Visitor.* **67**(5): 162–64.

Duniz M, Scheer PJ, Trojovsky A, Kaschnitz W, Kvas E and Macari S (1996) Changes in psychopathology of parents of NOFT (non-organic failure to thrive) infants during treatment. *European Child and Adolescent Psychiatry.* **5**(2): 93–100.

Gardner SL and Hagedorn MI (1991a) Physiologic sequelae of prematurity: the nurse practitioner's role. Feeding difficulties and growth failure (pathophysiology, cause, and data collection). Part 5. *Journal of Pediatric Health Care.* **5**(3): 122–34.

Gardner SL and Hagedorn MI (1991b) Physiologic sequelae of prematurity: the nurse practitioner's role. Feeding difficulties and growth failure (prevention, intervention, parent teaching, and complications). Part 6. *Journal of Pediatric Health Care.* **5**(6): 306–14.

Rosenthal SR, Sheppard JJ and Lotze M (1995) *Dysphagia and the Child with Developmental Disabilities.* Singular Publishing Group, California.

Index